ENEMA STORY

ENEMA STORY

by

Normane Cobbleson

This novel is a work of fiction. The characters, names, incidents, dialogue, and plot are the products of the author's imagination or are used fictitiously. Any resemblance to actual persons or institutions is purely coincidental

The author uses a pseudonym, and any resemblance to another person or persons is purely coincidental.

Copyright @ 2000 by Normane Cobbleson

All rights reserved. No part of this book may be reproduced, stored in a retrieval system, or transmitted by any means, electronic, mechanical, photocopying, recording, or otherwise, without the written permission of the author.

ISBN 1-58721-162-9

Copyright Protection Year 2000 By U.S. Common Law and Berne Convention

1st Books rev. 2/24/00

About The Book

Enema Story is adult fiction written primarily for those who judiciously take enemas or colonic irrigations based upon health or religious beliefs, or for sexual enhancement. Also, someone trying to understand why another takes them may find the story revealing. Of course, there is always room for the open minded and curious.

This novella is reality based and historically accurate. The world is divided on the subject, with those for and against enema use just as adamant. Since ancient Egyptian times, people have taken enemas: kings, queens, American presidents, the religious, and farmers, to name a few groups. The beloved Princess Diana, God rest her soul, was known to frequent a colonic irrigation clinic. One well-known American entertainer believes in taking coffee enemas to treat her depression. Only a statistician could estimate how many millions practice the therapy worldwide. Based upon hundreds of hours of study and discussions on the Internet, it would be safe to guess that most older users were given their first enema at the hands of a caring and loving mother during early childhood. Many doctors of a past era recommended the sensible use

of them to treat and prevent illness.

Although they are not fashionable today, full displays of enema equipment in drugstore windows and multi-page advertisements in major catalogues are etched in the author's memory. The end of the "golden age" of the enema generally correlates with the introduction of antibiotics, doctors' liability, and diminished interest in self-care. Much of the book is based upon information gleaned from Internet chats, where people are free to discuss intimate topics with anonymity.

Enema Story is about the life of a fictional character, Charlie Wisner. The time frame is from the late 1930s to the new millennium. The story details the enema and colonic irrigation aspects of the character's life from childhood through college and military service, then onto marriage. The novel is unusual because the subject matter has been considered taboo in recent years, and the focus of the story is on this aspect of Charlie's life. The story includes much about Charlie's sex life. His moral mind set developed during a time prior to the sexual revolution and widespread use of the birth-control pill. This narrow focus presented a challenge and produced an interesting approach to storytelling.

The author hopes readers will find the story to be interesting and entertaining, but an underlying purpose of *enema story* is to suggest to the enema user, who may feel isolated, that *he* or *she* is far from alone in their use. For example, I know that there are many who think that they are the only person who self-administered an enema as a child, but they should know that I have communicated with dozens of people who admit to giving themselves enemas as young children or teenagers. Although the author writes about intimate subjects in this book, it is done with the intent of telling a story about a human being with a good soul, and natural motives.

Note: This story is not to be used for the purpose of medical or health diagnosis or treatment, especially regarding the use of enemas or colonic irrigations. This is a work of fiction. Enemas and colonic irrigations are invasive bodily procedures, and there are potentially serious risks associated with them. Enemas and colonic irrigations should only be taken under supervision or approval of an appropriate and licensed health professional.

Table Of Contents

About The Book v

Main Street House 1

Water Street House 7

North Street House 25

The College Years 49

Soldier Boy 83

Enemates Forever 105

Your Story 123

About the Author 125

Main Street House

I have read in several places that around ten years old a child enters the "age of awareness." This may be true in my case because before age ten I remember only flashes of my life, similar to scenes taken from a movie. Although these scenes are relatively few, say, compared to the whole of my early childhood, each scene appears sharp, like glossy photos taken by an expert. The passing of almost six decades has not dulled those images. By the way, my name is Charlie Wisner.

I remember people rubbing my head, picking me up, hugging and kissing me. I can still feel those warm flannel pajamas on cold Colorado nights, and Mom tucking me into bed with a loving kiss. I remember playing without concerns or worries; I had a loving childhood. Other than the occasional fright caused by the hustle and bustle going on around me due to World War II, my memories are of feeling safe and loved. Because of the war, I hardly remember my father before I was eight years old, something he remedied later. His name was Edward Wisner. During my earliest years, my life centered around my mother, Mary, my five-year-older sister, Anna, and

whatever house we lived in. Anna and I were born in America, but our parents were born in Sweden. Among the most vivid and powerful of those memories are of my mother giving me enemas. The first one administered to me must have been when I was around the age of four, when I had pneumonia. Years later, I heard my mother, who was a nurse, comment to someone about giving me an enema during my bout of pneumonia at age four. From later conversations I also know that we moved from the Main Street house about the same time. The image of that first enema is brief. I remember lying on my belly on the kitchen table. For some reason, I see myself lying there naked, not unlike a tight-skinned wriggling little pig. My nine-year-old sister is standing on a kitchen chair, holding a red enema bag with a red hose fitted to the bottom side. I can still see Mother holding that black nozzle attached to the business end of the hose, and I remember Mother giving my sister instructions on holding the bag, feeling her holding me down firmly, and the unusual feeling of the nozzle sliding into my butt. The memory ends there.

The only other time I saw this red bag being used at the Main Street house was when I inadvertently walked in on my mother as she was douching in the bathtub. I stayed but

a few moments, but what I saw was indelibly imprinted into my brain. We were face to face as she lay naked with her back leaning up against the opposite end of the bathtub. Her feet were flat and legs raised at an angle and spread open, revealing a large area covered with hair. She held a large, curved nozzle in one hand. With the fingers of her other hand, she was spreading the flesh embedded in the hair. To my amazement, her fingers revealed something gaping and ugly, yet fascinating, even at my age. I knew girls were different than boys because they had long hair on their heads, acted differently, and played with dolls. Because my sister and I shared a bedroom, I saw her naked on several occasions, and knew little girls were smooth between their legs, quite different than I. But this event was a revelation. After that, I surmised that mothers were quite different than little sisters, not only above the waist, but below as well.

In character for my unperturbed mother, she calmly said, "Close the door, please go on and play; I will be out in a little bit." I quickly closed the door, feeling embarrassed, but enlightened.

I remember her coming out later, picking me up, giving me a kiss, as if to tell me everything was okay. Then we sat

down on the living room couch, and she said, "What you saw between my legs is called a vagina, and sometimes mothers wash out their vagina. It doesn't hurt. Now go ahead and play while I work on supper." It was as simple as that. My curiosity was satisfied for the time being.

Looking back, I wonder if that was the beginning of our extra-ordinary bond of trust. After all, I had seen my mother's most private parts, and she shared something very personal about herself. As it turned out, my mother and I could talk about anything, including what most people consider very private, and we did so without shame or embarrassment. Also, I could count on mother's being honest and telling me what I needed to know. Ever the nurse, she always called body parts by their proper name. I did not grow up with the implication that something was wrong with the private parts of the body because of the use of cute euphemisms. In turn, I was always honest with her.

From then on, I noticed enema syringes, probably because I knew what they were used for. Ours hung on the inside of the bathroom door. Mom usually hung her bathrobe on the same hook. Most homes that I visited had an enema bag and hose hanging somewhere, usually in the bathroom. So by the time our family moved out of the Main

Street house, the enema syringe was a common sight. In perspective, these flashes of memory added up to only a few minutes of my life on Main Street. However, as a small four-year-old boy, I had no idea how use of the home enema would influence my life.

Water Street House

Rather than continue paying rent, we moved to an affordable house on Water Street. A close friend and nurse, Fran Adams, told my mother about the house. Water Street was not far from where Fran lived. Plus, Fran was unmarried, liked children, and agreed to baby-sit for Mom when needed, and when she was available. As it turned out, Fran became like a second mother to me and sis. Mom and she loved to garden, and as Fran was in an apartment, they shared a "Victory Garden" planted on our property. I worked in the garden with them, which was mainly play. However, I did pull a few weeds now and then. We ate many meals together, and became like an extended family. Although Fran died years ago, I still miss her.

Everything went well for me until I started attending school. There was no established kindergarten system to prepare me for the first grade. I was the youngest child in my class of fifty, an immature five-year-old. In those days, children were required to enter school upon reaching the legal age, not when mature. Enlightened educators eventually learned that a child should start school when developmentally ready. I lacked the coordination for simple

coloring, something common for less mature children, especially little boys. It was not surprising that I was frustrated and struggled through the first grade. The teacher was new, and tried her best for me and the other fifty kids in my class, but she was not a miracle worker.

According to my mother, I had experienced some bowel discomfort since birth, but after starting school, I began having agonizing cramps that would put me on the floor, drawn up and crying in pain. Years later, I read that stress can cause problems in the gastrointestinal tract.

I would get a terrible nauseated feeling, accompanied by severe lower abdominal cramps. I needed to move my bowels, and would try, but straining yielded no results. Eventually, after long suffering, my bowels would move, but I would have a difficult, searing and constipated movement, followed by diarrhea. Moving the bowels always brought relief from the agonizing cramps. The doctor prescribed several remedies to be taken orally, but they tended to make the symptoms more acute.

We called our family practitioner, Dr. Bill. He, like many doctors of the era (and hundreds of years prior for that matter), believed that enema therapy could be useful. I remember Dr. Bill laying me down on his exam table. He

pushed, prodded and listened through his stethoscope. He asked Mother if I had been under any new stresses recently. Mother told him about my difficulties at school.

"He gets along well with the teachers and other children, but he has a hard time with the school work. He even has trouble coloring in outlines of figures."

"I see," Dr. Bill responded.

He told my mother, "I feel nothing abnormal in his abdomen. As he does not have appendicitis, I think we should try enemas. Enemas can be very dangerous if one has appendicitis. And, as you know, too many enemas can cause too much water to be absorbed into the bloodstream, causing an electrolyte imbalance, especially in children. I believe Charlie has a condition called spastic colon. However, it is foolish to continue to irritate the entire gastrointestinal tract when only the last few feet need treatment. Go ahead and give him an enema when he has acute cramping and can't move his bowels. An enema is safe, quick and effective. It will be easier as you have been trained to give them. Mrs. Wisner, I know you are experienced, but I have suggestions concerning the enema. Heat the water to about body temperature and mix in a little Castile soap until the water is cloudy, not sudsy; too much

soap unduly irritates the colon. Gently push some Vaseline into his rectum before starting. This will help prevent irritation from the soap and nozzle abrasion. If at all possible, have him hold it a few minutes. It may help to massage his belly. I can't stress enough the importance of giving the enema at low pressure, with slow, gentle delivery, as lovingly as possible. It's important to not traumatize Charlie. If the enema is delivered with the bag high above his anus, the enema will be delivered harshly, and Charlie will resist future enemas. Our goal is to keep him as relaxed as possible. This makes the enema easier to take and more effective. It's really an opportunity to develop a trusting relationship between you and your child. With care, this will be very beneficial, and a mostly pleasant experience for Charlie. The emotional aspect of an enema is as important as the mechanics. Here are some printed instructions to follow. Let's see how this works for him.

"We may have to do more invasive tests, but I don't want to put him through all of that unnecessarily. Call and let me know how he does and we'll go from there."

He went on, "Maybe a tutor will help with his school work, and at the same time lower his stress level. Spastic

colon seems to be caused or made worse by stress. We still have a lot to learn about this condition. But if he has spastic colon, the good news is that his large bowel will appear normal, and it is not a life-threatening disease."

Of course I was all ears. I knew what an enema was, and now that I was older, the thought of getting one was scary indeed.

It was not long before I was sent home from school in the early afternoon with severe abdominal cramps. By the time I got home I was doubled up in pain, and would have submitted to almost anything that would stop the sickening agony. Mom picked me up, and took me to the toilet to see if I could move my bowels. After straining and straining, the only result was more sickening cramps and sweats.

To this day, I can remember Mother sitting on the edge of the bathtub facing me as I sat on the toilet. She looked me straight in the eyes and said, "Charlie, you need help. This is the time to try taking an enema as Dr. Bill suggested. I think it will make you feel much better. Okay?"

I nodded yes. I was sweating profusely and in misery.

"Charlie, I'm not going to surprise you with anything, and I'll let you know each step of the way what I'm doing.

You know, Charlie, I always tell you the truth."

She got up and took the enema bag down from the hook on the bathroom door, and she sat back down in front of me.

"Charlie, I am going to lay a board down lengthwise across the top of the tub. I'll lay you down on top of the board for the enema. I'm going to hang a bag of warm, soapy water on the rack in front of you. Then you can take a place lying down on a towel I've put over the board. I'll wash your bottom with warm soap and water and put some Vaseline in your rectum with my finger so that the nozzle will go in easily. None of this will hurt. See this clamp? After the nozzle is inside your rectum, I'll click open this clamp, and let the water go inside of you. You will feel it running in, and it will be pleasant and warm. At some point you'll feel a cramp. Tell me when you do. If it hurts too bad, I will stop the water. When you have to go to the toilet real bad, let me know and I will set you on it. When done, this should make you feel much better.

"Now get ready for bed while I go to the kitchen and fix the enema -okay?"

I nodded yes.

She hugged me and gave me a kiss. She then said,

"Now go on. I won't be long. Everything will be okay." Mother had always been truthful with me, but I was still scared.

I could hear the rattle of pots and pans as she retrieved one to warm the water in. This would be a familiar sound over the years to come, a signal that Mother might be preparing an enema for me or my sister, or sometimes for herself or for Dad.

I dutifully took off my school clothes, put on my pajamas, climbed into bed, and waited anxiously. In a short while I saw her walk across the hall into the bathroom with the half full, but bulging enema bag. In a few minutes she came into my bedroom. Although I was six years old by now and getting bigger, she walked over to my bed and picked me up as easily as if I were a feather. She said, "Come here, baby, we are going to make you feel better."

As she carried me to the bathroom, I'm sure she could feel my sobbing. I tried to hide my tears, but she had to see them. I think the tears were caused as much by fatigue and stress due to the pain, as fear of the enema. Upon entering the bathroom, I could see the red bag suspended from the towel rack over the tub, and I could smell the odor of Castile soap. A little of the soapy water had slushed down

over the side of it. The red hose with the black nozzle was left curled over the bag. Mom hugged and kissed me before helping me onto the toweled board. I could not help but notice that her eyes were moist with tears. After laying me down, she stroked my brow and whispered in my ear, "You'll be fine."

She gently pulled off my pajama bottoms and rolled me onto my left side, with my left leg slightly bent. Then she pulled my right leg, the top leg, up toward my stomach, until it was well flexed. I remember this as it were happening today. She washed my bottom and gently dried me off.

She put on a rubber glove, opened the nearby jar of Vaseline, and said, "Now relax, Charlie, we need to put some lubrication in your rectum so the nozzle will go in easily and not hurt.

I could feel her greased finger gently massaging around the opening in my butt, then she pushed against my anus. She waited briefly. It seemed to relax on its own. "Charlie, push down like you are trying to move your bowels."

As I pushed down, I could feel my rectum "swallow" her finger, as if invited. She entered, rotated her finger in each direction, then gently withdrew it.

"Now, that wasn't so bad, was it?"

I nodded in agreement.

I did not understand why at the time, but it felt good to have my rectum lubricated. Years later, I realized that she lubricated my rectum to avoid abrasion and irritation of the delicate membrane lining when inserting the nozzle and injecting the solution. In addition to all of the loving and gentle kindness I was receiving, I discovered that one of the pleasures of a properly given enema was the anal-rectal preparation, an area that teemed with sensual nerves, now fully awakened within me.

Mom reached up toward the enema bag and took down the nozzle end of the hose. I heard her click open the clamp. Water ran out into the tub.

"We have to let some water run through the hose to clear out air in the line. If I let the air go inside you, it will cause additional cramping." With that done, she closed the clamp with a sharp click.

"This has not been so bad, has it?"

I somehow knew a defining moment was about to occur.

"Bear down just a little bit, and I will slide this into your rectum ever so easily. Now you hardly felt that, did

you?"

I nodded in agreement.

What little I felt was pleasurable. Mother held the nozzle in me with her right hand, and with her left began to lightly massage my buttocks and back, in a manner that was relaxing. She reached over and massaged my belly a bit more vigorously.

"Relax, Charlie, relax."

Mother had followed the doctor's instructions closely, and so far the results were gratifying for both of us. I was calm and doing well, but she knew the acid test was coming up.

"We are going to start now," she announced, and she opened the clamp with a definite click.

Mother kept one hand on the nozzle and the other firmly on my buttocks. When the surge of warm water hit my innards, my buttocks moved up with a quick jerk, then relaxed. Thinking back, I remember it feeling like a fast-flowing river inside of me. It was warm and pleasant.

Then suddenly, I said, "Mama, I have to potty bad."

Mother closed the clamp, shutting off the flow.

"Is that better, Charlie?"

She wanted to see if it was just a passing cramp, but I

had an overpowering need to expel. She withdrew the nozzle. She picked me up and swung me over onto the toilet. She left me to finish in private. I immediately eliminated the enema. I felt like my insides were pouring out. Even now, I remember the relief being tremendous. Over time, I learned that Mom put a small amount of peppermint in the enema water. She said this helped remove gas in my bowels and made the air less odoriferous.

After I finished and cared for myself, Mother came back in and asked, "Can you stand up, Charlie?"

"Yes, Mama."

"Bend over the tub onto the board and I will wash your bottom."

The warm water felt good. I felt weak, but much better. After washing me, she helped me step back into my pajama bottoms. She carried me to back to my bed. She hugged and kissed me, then told me how brave I was, and how well I had done. She tucked me in under the covers, where I soon fell into a calm sleep. The next thing I remember is being awakened for supper. I was served my supper in bed and allowed full rest until morning. I heard Mother call the doctor and tell him of our success.

The next morning Mother massaged my belly; it felt

soft and supple to our touch. The pain and soreness were gone. I felt better than I could ever remember. I was ready to go back to school. Before this, I was usually home sick for days. This was a remarkable improvement over the past, and for whatever reason, my cramps occurred less frequently after starting to take the enemas. Sometimes I would need another enema within a week, but usually I would go a month or two before needing another.

Mom found a tutor who helped me to keep up with my school work. She also helped me to have many small successes needed to build my confidence. Mom later said that the tutor helped lessen my stress at school, and in turn lessened my "tummy problem," just as the doctor predicted.

"Tummy problem" was the only medical euphemism I heard my mother use. I think she used it rather than *spastic colon* because of the difficulty of explaining that terminology to other six-year-old children as to why I could not come out and play. My friends could all understand "tummy problem." Thus, the first enema I had as a "big boy" was a successful treatment for my condition, and provided a foundation for my future care. Fortunately, I was not traumatized, so I did not fear this treatment. I could tolerate the mild discomforts that came along with

the therapy because the benefit was so great, and for the most part, pleasant. The treatments also established a special bond of trust between me and my mother. By the time I reached the summer of my sixth year, I was not afraid to ask for an enema when I felt the onset of colon cramps.

Although I was quite shy, I was not embarrassed when Mother showed Fran how she gave me an enema. Fran was like a second mother to me, and besides, this is what nurses did. After Fran started giving me enemas in Mother's absence, she and I developed that same trusting bond.

As I grew older, I was aware that Mother and Fran gave each other enemas when they were ill. They also believed in the period use of enema therapy to prevent illness. We all received them with the change of seasons as a health measure. I could always tell when one of them needed an enema between seasons because one would say, "I need a good cleaning out. Do you have some time?"

Sis would get one occasionally when she stayed home from school with a cold or was constipated, but most of her enemas were the seasonal ones. My sister was more outspoken than I, and she told her friends that she liked getting them.

An enema syringe was on the list of recommended medical supplies for home medicine chests, so when sis went away to college, Mother packed one among her home supplies.

The war finally ended, and Dad was home. He took me with him every chance he could. We became great friends. Mom gave him enemas also when needed.

Dad gave me only one. I wanted to go out and play baseball with friends one day, but Mom thought I needed to stay in because I had a bad cold. Mom believed in an enema and bed rest for colds. She still feared, as in the pre-antibiotic days, that a cold could turn into a secondary bacterial infection and cause pneumonia, which was the leading cause of death at the time. I was particularly at risk for that illness anyway. All of my grandparents had died of either tuberculosis or pneumonia. As mentioned earlier, I had pneumonia at age four. At the present time, however, I was strongly resisting having to stay inside. Dad was home that day, and to my surprise, he stepped in and took charge, but I continued to resist and struggle. I was embarrassed about the idea of Dad's giving me an enema. I had worked myself into a corner. After I received a brisk swat on my bare butt, I settled down, and he give me the enema, and

saw to it that I stayed in bed. It was at that point, I understood that he was not only my friend, but my dad as well. I further understood that he and mother worked together as a team. Instinctively, I knew he loved me as well. After the swat on the butt, he became as loving as my mother. Somehow seeing this side of my dad was fortunate. Again, the enema use helped provide a bond between us.

In those days most girls married just after high school, and many mothers considered it a duty to teach their daughters how to give enemas, some by using a younger sibling as the patient. Indeed, my sister gave me an enema under the supervision of my mother when I was eleven years old. My sister was sixteen at the time. I did not like the idea, but did not complain because I needed relief from my cramps. The truth is, she did a good job. She had always mothered me anyway, and I knew she would never hurt me. I would have let her give me another one in an emergency, but Mother or Fran was always around when I needed one.

Not long after sis gave me the enema, she and one of her friends, Brenda, started giving each other enemas when needed, rather than receive them from their mothers. Both

mothers agreed that it was okay as long as they limited their use so as not to develop an enema habit.

I was embarrassed when I heard sis tell Brenda how she first learned to give an enema. Brenda noticed I was embarrassed. She walked over and got down on one knee and said, "It's okay, Charlie. I know you have needed a lot of enemas. You can't help it. I'll help you if you are ever in trouble. I won't tell anyone." With that she gave me a motherly hug. Brenda never gave me an enema, but after that incident I felt close to her.

Other than receiving more enemas than most of my friends because of my spastic colon, I lived a normal little boy's life. In many ways my childhood was idyllic. I had lots of love at home, as well as from neighbors, teachers, and friends. As to my spastic colon, I slowly learned more about the condition as it applied to me. Each new bit of useful information enabled me to feel better.

The decade of the forties was ending. My parents began sharing in the growing affluence of middle-class America. They built a new house. Fran found a husband and moved into a house with him. Fortunately for me, Fran lived only a few blocks from us. We all remained close friends, and I could count on Fran should I need help in any way. Fran's

husband understood my condition and that his wife had nursing duties regarding me. He never interfered or made me feel embarrassed.

After living in our new house for about a year, I had passed the "age of awareness," and was now eleven. I noticed growth of new body hair, but did not know that signaled puberty as well.

Our new house was on North Street. Although my need for enemas was less frequent, a new aspect of the enema entered my life, quite by surprise.

North Street House

We had not lived long on North Street when I came into the house on a hot summer day in 1950, just before my twelfth birthday. I had been playing baseball for several hours out in the hot sun. I was exhausted from the heat, gulped down a couple of glasses of water, turned on the fans, and sat down, feeling lethargic. Mother and Dad were off with my sister to a baton-twirling contest and would not be home for several hours. I felt cramps and needed to move my bowels, so I went to the toilet, with no results. I knew from past experience my cramps would only get worse, and eventually Mother or Fran would have to give me an enema. I was reminded of this as I sat on the toilet and looked at the bathroom door, upon which hung our enema syringe. In those days they all looked about the same. They varied in size, but all were red, with usually an open top, and a black nozzle of some sort attached to the business end of a red hose. Some were closed at the top and could double as hot water bottles. All had a silver metal clamp to stop and start the flow of solution from the bag. Mom used the adult rectal nozzle because it had long been more comfortable to insert than the slightly smaller

one for infants.

Most of my friends had similar enema apparatus hanging somewhere in their houses, usually on the inside bathroom door. We all knew that each of us was occasionally given enemas, but we did not talk about it much.

I look back now and realize I was badly dehydrated that day, not to mention plagued by my longtime problem of spastic colon. I should have drunk the water, and more of it, earlier, rather than later, but children put off things while enjoying their play. Plus, there wasn't air conditioning to retreat to during the heat of the summer.

From age six on, the sight of that red enema bag gave me more and more of a strange, but good feeling that I liked. Over the years, I felt the urge to give myself an enema for reasons I could not explain.

Before you knew it, I would be swishing a bar of Castile soap around in a two-quart pot of warm water, just as I had seen my mother do, determined to give myself an enema that very day. My hands trembled with excitement and fear. With some spillage into the kitchen sink, I filled the bag with the soapy solution. I decided to take it in the bathtub, so I hung the bag on the faucet above the drain. I

opened the clamp to allow some water to run into the tub to let the air out of the hose, as I had seen my mother do so many times. Then I put a generous amount of Vaseline on the adult rectal nozzle, and curled the hose around the faucet. Just looking at the bulging bag gave me a feeling of shortness of breath, caused by a strange force deep within my pelvis.

I lay a towel down on the bottom of the cold tub, then nervously stripped off my few clothes, and climbed into the bathtub. I lay on my back with feet flat, legs flexed with knees raised. I parted my legs, reached for the hose, raised my butt a bit, and then slowly inserted the glistening black nozzle into my waiting rectum, sliding it past countless sensuous nerves, causing what I now know as a prostate spasm. The prostate was unknown to me at the time, and it would be decades later before I would hear this marvelous gland described as the male G spot.

I can remember clicking open the metal clamp as if it were just moments ago; I still feel a deep genital response from that memory, all these decades later. The feeling of the gush of water that entered my hinder parts is like no other I can describe, almost like a non-electric current. Something more than an enema was taking place. Yes, I

was filling my colon with warm, soapy water, but with the heat and pressure came a building agony, unlike a cramp, something I could not stop. It was a wonderful agony, and it grew ever more rapidly. I would not have wanted to stop, even if I could, though it was mysteriously taking my breath. It was overwhelming, but welcomed. Suddenly, my body began to stiffen, became rigid, then started to spasm. I involuntarily released the nozzle and braced my hands against the floor of the tub. My head was thrust back, and I cried out for relief. Agonizing relief came in strong spasmodic spurts, which slowly weakened. Then my body fell into a relaxed, but breathless state.

I do not know how much time passed before I noticed the white liquid on my face and belly, or noticed that I had been soaked by the nozzle that had escaped my innards, the bag now drained.

When my mind and eyes glazed over, I had lost track of time. Now resolved, and breath regained, I looked down and studied my male member slowly falling from a rigid state. How comedic my mound must have looked, with the thin wisp of pubic hair soaked down, making me look more like a baby than the man I wanted to be. No sooner had I gotten relaxed than I began to cramp from the part of the

enema I had injected. I quickly picked up my wet body and sat on the toilet to allow the enema to do its job, a second wonderful relief that brought on a feeling of lightness, well-being, and a healthy glow.

In my ignorance I thought the white stuff was some of the soapy enema that somehow made its way through my system and passed out through my child-sized penis. Little did I understand what happened that day, but I soon learned. I know one thing: My first ejaculation, albeit spontaneous, came at the same time as my first self-administered enema. This left a wonderful and unforgettable imprint upon me. What a blessing for these two great events to come together at the same time, events that I am able to enjoy to this day, much to my health and happiness as a normal, but blessed adult.

About a week later, I was standing up urinating into that same toilet. As most men and boys do, I stroked myself a couple of times after finishing, but this time those same agonizing, but wonderful feelings overwhelmed me again. I could not stop stroking. My body became rigid, my head was down, then was thrust back, and soon relief came again in strong spurts. I fell against the bathroom wall in breathless resolution. I had unknowingly masturbated for

the first time. I did not understand what happened, but I knew it was not soap from an enema that I had spattered about. I knew one thing, I liked it, and it would became a regular part of my life.

Soon after that, I would frequently wake up in the morning, wet, experiencing those same feelings at the end of an erotic dream. A "wet dream" is a gift from God, I think, being without the accompanying guilt, no matter the mess. Because I knew so little of erotica, I have always wondered where those erotic visions came from. Again, God seems to provide what we need.

I began to hear rumors from other boys, rumors that "beating off," "jacking off," or "pounding your pud" could cause insanity, blindness, and hair to grow on the palms of your hands. Of course, I still could not stop doing it. Again, it would be the enema that indirectly saved me from these needless worries.

As I entered my teens, I was still comfortable with the idea of Mother or Fran giving me enemas when I was sick or having a spastic colon attack. It was a routine. I was made to feel comfortable when pubic hair started to appear, and I was proud that I was finally going to look like every other male, especially my dad. Fran told me that it was a

sign that I was beginning to be a man. I had occasional erections during enemas, but that had always been, and I understood that it was a normal reaction.

By now I was in the eighth grade. One day I was sick, and the school called Fran because she was the backup contact that day. Mom left word for them to call Fran in case of an emergency. Mom had a special-duty nursing job, so Fran picked me up from school. I was in agony with cramps, so Fran took me home, and told me to undress while she prepared the remedy.

I was in such pain, she expedited the process by suspending the bag from the towel rack in the bathroom, and had me get into the knee-chest position on the floor. She sat on the toilet, facing my raised rear. When she lubricated my rectum with her gloved index finger, I felt a spasm.

For some time now Mom and Fran used a 20-inch-long colon tube to deliver my enemas. The red rubber tube was pressed onto the adult rectal nozzle on one end. It was about the diameter of a pencil, with an opening in the end, and sort of a slitted hole on the side. As the water was injected the tube was threaded gently, but deeply, into my bowel. They were both nurses and knew how to safely

insert the tube. With the tube I could be filled more completely and comfortably before the water would come back into the rectum under pressure. Once there were pressure on my rectum, I would have a strong urge to empty my bowels. After I grew older, Mom and Fran said they gave me high enemas for a deeper cleansing.

However, on this occasion Fran opened the clamp, and when the warm water and pressure hit my innards, I began to experience a strong orgasm. Although it was unusual for me, I had not masturbated for several days, and I was biologically ready for an emission, despite my cramps. I tried to stop the orgasm, but it was impossible.

To Fran, there could not have been any doubt as to what was happening. I moaned involuntarily, but loudly. I became breathless, and the colon tube waved in my rectum with each prostate spasm. I soon spurted semen along the floor.

"It's okay, Charlie, this sometimes happens during enemas. I think we should finish, if you can."

I weakly said, "Okay." I could not help what happened, but I was embarrassed nonetheless.

Fran put her hand on my back and buttocks, and said, "Relax now."

I took the rest of the enema with ease. I was very relaxed after ejaculating.

After the warm water ran in, she gently snaked out the colon tube, and helped me to the nearby bedroom, where I lay down on a towel she had spread on the bed. Fran then began to massage my belly. Clear fluid was still oozing from my penis. She noticed tears in my eyes. I was so embarrassed. She had tears in her eyes as well. She bent over and kissed me above my brow, and said, "I love you, Charlie."

After a while I needed to expel. She helped me up and I went to the bathroom, where I voided the enema, moved my bowels and felt much better.

Fran called my mother and told her what happened, and that she thought this was an auspicious time to explain sex to me, but first she wanted my mother's permission.

"Of course, Fran, you are like a mother to him. Be sure to explain that masturbation is okay and that everyone does it. It's God's way of providing natural relief. I don't want him to fear all those myths about going insane and all. He should know that people masturbate, some during all of their lives."

Fran went back to the bathroom, and through the closed

door, she told me to put on my pajamas when I was done. When I came back into the living room, she explained to me that she had called my mother and told her I was fine, but that I had an ejaculation during my enema.

"Your mother and I agreed that now might be a good opportunity to explain about sex. Charlie, come over and sit next to me." Fran put her arms around me and hugged me. I could feel her sobbing. I could tell that she had been moved by what had happened.

Over the next three hours we talked about sex from A to Z, with great emphasis on responsibility, consideration, and love, in addition to the mechanics. I would never worry about masturbating again. I had been assured by my mother and Fran that it was a normal and natural thing to do, although something to be done in private. In fact, it became a useful activity for the rest of my life, especially prior to my marriage. It allowed me to be the gentleman my family expected me to be. Many times, I masturbated before a date to control my passions. Even at that, many times I repeated after a date. I knew this was a much better way to deal with my sensual needs. I understood why this was better than leading a promiscuous life. I enjoyed hot dates, without the risks of causing a pregnancy or

contracting a sexually transmitted disease.

We also talked about the sensuous and sexual side of enemas experienced by some persons in a relaxed state. (A few years later I discovered that if pain, discomfort, and embarrassment composed the total experience, many would fear, even hate receiving enemas.)

I also learned during the talk about sex that because of our wonderful anatomy, it was normal to experience sensual feelings during a well-administered enema, and how some of those feelings might become sexual at this stage of my development called *puberty*. This was the first time I heard the word *puberty*. Fran explained that regardless of how good the enema felt, it must always be used responsibly and with self-discipline. Keeping this in mind, the enema could remain a beneficial therapy, while being a pleasant experience. I remember that Mom and Fran repeatedly stressed health factors as the prime reason for taking enemas.

I remember Fran saying, "For those who know how to use them, enemas are like chocolate candy. A little bit is very good, but too much may be harmful."

Fran also explained the role of the prostate gland and promised to show me where the gland was the next time

she prepared me for an enema. She explained where the small chestnut-sized gland was located, and all she had to do to touch it was to insert her finger just a little deeper while lubricating my rectum. She kept her promise. The next time she pre-lubricated my rectum for an enema, she briefly touched it to show me exactly where it was. After that, I fully understood its sexual role. Just a brief touching of this gland gave me the feeling I was going to ejaculate.

As she touched the gland she said, "Did you feel that?"

I could not help but immediately respond with a gasping, "Oh yes!"

I knew that if she touched my gland more than briefly I would have an orgasm. It was not difficult to understand how it was possible to experience an orgasm while having an enema. The mechanical action of the warm water pressuring the prostate, not to mention the added stimulation to anal and genital nerves, made things very clear, even for a thirteen-year-old.

Fran went on, saying, "Charlie, I hope you might also understand that when you are taking enemas primarily for health reasons, you should not feel guilty concerning any good feelings or responses. I take one occasionally just to feel good and relieve stress, and that is reason enough to

take one. But it is important not to take so many enemas that the colon becomes lazy and dependent upon them to move your bowels. Also, there is good stuff in there called intestinal flora. If you are taking enemas all the time, the flora never get a chance to be reestablished."

I did not remember all of this verbatim or fully understand then, but it was discussed in part over the years that followed, the result of an open and loving family atmosphere.

It was during that same long revelation that I learned that my mother and Fran also believed in the appropriate use of enemas based upon ancient religious teachings, dating back to the time of Christ. They believed that Jesus was a Jewish Essene, and they followed many of the teachings found in the *Essene Gospel of Peace*. Of course, Mom's and Fran's beliefs greatly influenced me. As I grew older many of those teachings made sense to me.

After such a personal discussion with Fran that memorable day, I felt free to talk with her about anything. She indeed was a second mother to me. Fran told My mother about "the talk," and Mother likely told Dad. This helped form the trusting bond among all of us. We all seemed comfortable knowing that I did not live in

ignorance of sex. In fact, the parts of "the talk" about enemas were insignificant compared with what I learned about how babies came about, love, responsibility, and how I should respect the opposite gender. "The talk" became part of the great foundation of my future as a sexual human being, not to mention how helpful it was to me as a virile teenager. I didn't grow up confused about sex, normal sensuous feelings, God, religion, church, or responsibility. "The talk," and the many that followed between me and Mom, Dad, and Fran, made me one of the luckiest children alive. To this day, I believe it was the properly handled intimacy associated with giving of the enema that was crucial in my life on so many fronts. It provided the vehicle that introduced me, by happenstance, to other difficult and intimate subjects. I'm sure my loved ones may well have found other vehicles, but mine turned out to be the enema.

Based upon my reading, listening and Internet chats, most parents of the past stopped giving their boys enemas when they reached puberty. Typically, they gave their girls enemas until a bit later in life. Some taught their children to self-administer enemas. One man told me that, when he was nine, his mother prepared the enema and handed it to

him through the bathroom door for him to give to himself. I have read that many parents stop this therapy because of the obvious sexual component involved. The appearance of pubic hair, erections, visible flow of fluids, etc. causes embarrassment to child and parent, if not explained at the right time. Rather than looking at this as an opportunity to further bond with their child, they are unwilling or unable to "deal with" the situation. It was fortuitous that I still needed enemas because they were the only thing my family knew of that was effective for treating my spastic colon. I also think I needed them for general health reasons.

I have read that some proponents of enema use within the alternative medicine community believe that parents stop this practice when their children might need them most, especially in light of the questionable diet many teenagers have.

There is great need for sensitivity when giving an enema, but this is easier said than done. Most children did not have the advantage that I had of trained nurses giving me the therapy. Doctors and nurses develop a discipline regarding their sexual feelings when dealing with the naked body. They approach intimate treatments with objectivity, and they are usually ethical, caring and effective in their

professional duties. This is sometimes difficult for an untrained parent. Even if the professional has a sexual response while treating a patient, they do not let it interfere with their duties. They are also trained to overcome embarrassment for the good of their patient.

Except for an occasional self-administered enema, I continued getting them from Mom and Fran through my teens. I preferred Fran giving them to me because I continued to ejaculate spontaneously with more frequency as I got older. There must be some truth in what I have read, that males reach their sexual peak in the late teens. With the knowledge this may happen, I masturbated just prior to Mother's giving me an enema, if I felt the slightest biological need. However, if it had happened, I know we would have dealt with it.

I discovered something interesting while listening and chatting on the Net. Many, as children, continued to complain about getting enemas long after they found them pleasurable. Many felt they needed to keep up the appearance of complaint rather than pleasure. To their regret, their mothers stopped giving them because of the complaining. Many said they also enjoyed the caring attention, and the sense of well being they experienced after

each enema. These regrets were especially true among the many children whose mothers stopped this practice at the child's puberty.

Over the years that followed, I had what one would call a normal teenage life, except that I did not have many of the rebellion problems many teenagers had. There are people who believe that enemas have a calming, personality sweetening effect, not to mention stress relieving. Well, that seems to be the case with me. Enemas give me a sense of well-being, and always made me want to be loving, rather than aggressive.

It would be after my sixteenth birthday when I discovered, first-hand, why some people spoke of dreading enemas. I had been playing basketball after school when I developed a terrific pain in my right side. The pain was different than my usual spastic colon pain. Mother, in her wisdom, took me to Dr. Bill to check it out, and he diagnosed me as having appendicitis. By late evening a surgeon had removed my inflamed appendix, which was about to burst. It was fortunate that my mother did not give me an enema on this occasion. According to what I have read and heard, the pressure from an enema could have ruptured my appendix, spilling poison into my abdominal

cavity. A ruptured appendix could have been fatal!

This was my first stay in a hospital, and it turned out to be a memory from hell. To begin with, my nurse had just come in on a change of shift and neglected any notations from the previous shift. She thought the nurse from the prior shift had given me pain medication after the surgery. I suffered needlessly for hours. The nurse informed my mother that "I was just being a baby." Finally, in the wee hours of the morning, Mom called the doctor, and he straightened things out.

The next problem was that I could not urinate. For some reason, my bladder had been paralyzed by the spinal anaesthesia. It was two days before my bladder began to function normally. In the meantime, I had to be catheterized. The doctor came to my bed and began the procedure by encircling my penis with white towels. He tried and tried to get the catheter tube to go into my penis. Finally, the doctor angrily told the nurse, "This catheter is too big. After all, he is not a grown man." As all males will do, I compared my penis size to my fellow man. Many males do this during early sexual exploration. I was far too modest to participate in such things as "circle jerks," or mutual masturbation, and the like. My first look at other

males my age came in seventh-grade gym class. By age sixteen, I realized that I was not going to be "well-endowed," and would be average size at best. It would be a long time before I realized that things such as penis and female breast size were of little importance in the overall scheme of things, and that my sexual drive, sensitivity toward others, and my heart and soul were possessions to be cherished, far more than an extra few inches of penis size.

I waited for the nurse to get another catheter while my sore penis stuck up out of a field of clean towels. She finally returned, and this time the doctor was able to easily thread the new and smaller catheter tube through my penis and into my bladder. The relief was instantaneous. This had to be done for a couple days until my bladder began to function normally again. This was extremely humiliating for me as a sixteen-year-old; first, to be called a baby, and then having my relatively small penis size announced to my roommates.

On the third day a nurse's aide came in and said, "How are you, Charlie? You know my son Billy from school. I'm here to give you an enema. Don't worry; Billy gets them, too."

Billy had asked me one time why I missed school the day before. I told him I had a "tummy problem." Billy replied, "I get an enema for that; I hate getting enemas." At the time I didn't understand why he felt that way, but I soon would.

The nurse set a white enamel can on my bed-side stand. The can was full of sudsy water. She cranked the stand up as high as it would go. Attached to the can was a red, ribbed, rubber hose with a silver clamp near the opposite end of the can. I watched her glob on lots of petroleum jelly over the end of the blunt end of the enema hose. I wondered where the nozzle was. Without pulling the privacy drapes, she told me to lie on my left side. She pulled open my gown, exposing my bare bottom to her and my two roommates. She told me to bear down, then shoved the blunt end of the hose up my rectum. She never pre-lubricated me, nor did she use a nozzle.

It hurt as she shoved the hose in, not to mention my total humiliation. She said, "I'm starting it now. Take deep breaths in. That will help pull the enema in." I knew how to breathe in as Mom and Fran had taught me to do this long ago. The water was hot, rather than pleasantly warm. The soapy water was strong and burned my now-

abraded rectum. I started to cramp and I asked her to stop.

"You're okay," she said.

Not wanting to appear to be a baby, I tried to hold on. I looked down at my rapidly expanding belly. It was still orange from the antiseptic pre-incision wash. My large incision was still held together by many ugly stitches. I was now begging her to stop.

"I'm going to bust! STOP, OH PLEASE, STOP!"

I continued to beg, but she only stopped when the can gurgled empty. Then she withdrew the ribbed hose from my burning rear. Though sixteen, I was in tears and sobbing profusely. However, I was grateful when she shoved a bedpan under me. I did not care who was watching by then. As I expelled, I gratefully watched my orange and stitched abdomen recede. My butt burned for hours after.

It was hard to believe that this was the same place where my mother worked from time to time. From my experience, there was nothing loving and caring about this place. This was not what I was used to.

Although still fearing I would be called a baby, I complained to my mother. She contacted the doctor and he arranged for me to go home immediately. He said, "Take

him home where he can be cared for by a real nurse."

Recuperation from appendicitis was much slower in those days. I was out of school a couple of weeks. Because of the effects of the anaesthesia and the heavy doses of antibiotics, it took a few more enemas before my normal bowel function returned, but they were given to me by the best nurse in the country, my Mother. My faith in using enemas was restored.

However, after the hospital enema, I could understand why Billy dreaded them, and how enemas could be so emotionally, if not physically traumatic. If that hospital enema had been my first, I would have hated and resisted them forever, just as our family doctor had cautioned my mother back when I was in the first grade. Instead, I believe enemas helped me to grow up with a healthy awareness of my body, and for its proper care.

My spastic colon condition and other health beliefs were the reasons why Mom and Fran continued to give me enemas through my

high school years. But had it not been for the strong and trusting bond between us, I would not have had the advantage of their help. Like multitudes of others, I would have retreated to the loveless burden of self-care. I could

not have tolerated the added and unnecessary pain and embarrassment that my friend Billy suffered at the hands of his own mother.

The time eventually arrives when children grow up and leave their homes for various reasons. During the mid-1950s, most people married soon after completing high school. Virtually all physically-fit males went into military service or continued with their schooling. What did I do?

The College Years

A very small percentage of children attended college during the mid-1950s, but from childhood it was understood that I would be attending college one day. I chose a major state university miles away from home. Although Fran or Mom could give me an enema when I was home on vacation, they were not available to help most of the time. I had self-administered enemas on a few occasions before moving on to college, but this was the beginning of a long period of mostly giving them to myself. All these years later, I realize that there must have been plenty of girls at school who were of my same background and who would have helped me. Many would have appreciated my help as well. Again, because I was so modest, I did not look for "enema compatibility" in girls, let alone in my male friends. Of course, most people were as modest as I concerning such intimate subjects, but I erroneously believed that enema use was always an unmanly subject to mention to others.

Although females do not have a prostate gland, I understood that their bodies abound with sensuous nerves which generate powerful orgasms, with both anal and

clitoral stimulation. Knowing what I know now, I could have found compatible enemates. Based upon my recent Internet chats, it was a rare person of that era who realized that opposite-gender enemates were so plentiful. Therefore, few consciously found and married enemates, many to their regret. Many spouses spend their married lives as closet enema users. I have found cases where both partners were closet users, and did not know about their mate's same need for years. Others somehow achieved a level of communication regarding their enema use after marriage. These people are among the more fortunate to have married an open-minded partner, especially if their partner was negatively potty trained, which reinforced the belief that their privates were nasty or forbidden territory. Unfortunately, a significant number marry persons who were traumatized by experiences with enemas. They have a tendency to belittle their spouses and force them to hide their behavior. Of course, a good number stumble into marriage, only to find they have married an enemate.

I found self-administration a poor second choice compared with being given an enema by a caring person. When given, I can avail myself of more efficient positions that are not feasible solo, such as the knee-chest, or on the

back with hips raised by pillows. Also, I can relax much more when someone else does the work. The hands are then free to self-massage the abdomen. It is more comfortable because the giver can monitor and change solution pressure and flow by changing bag height, and safely control the nozzle position. The greatest advantage, however, may be the caring love shown to the receiver. We all need loving and encouraging words. Such care also helps the receiver get through uncomfortable moments that are inevitably experienced. Although the enema is a very private and intimate procedure, we all need intimacy under trusting and discreet conditions. I have found the enema a good way to help fulfill that need as well. But of course, I believed, and still do, that a carefully and appropriately self-administered enema is better than none.

For the enema user a college dorm room with a roommate provided little privacy. My roommate may have been willing to help me had I been brave enough to ask, but there was a growing silence concerning enemas, and I did not want to risk possible ridicule by the uninformed. Besides, I did not know much about these strangers with whom I was suddenly living.

Like my sister, I packed an enema bag to take to

college. Based upon my sister's experience, Mother also instructed me how to use the much smaller bulb syringe. She told me that I may find it helpful to self-inject a bulb full of warm water when I had acute attacks when the privacy for a full-fledged enema was not available. The bulb syringe was comparatively easy to fill in privacy. All I needed was to be alone in my room or in the large common bathroom. The bulb syringe was easy to store in a secret place before and after use. I could even inject the water in a bathroom stall if I did not have privacy in my own room. Mom felt the full enema would serve me better, but use of the bulb syringe could be helpful in emergencies. She understood my shyness outside of the family.

On several occasions during that first year I was able to take a quick bulb enema in my room while my roommate was gone to class. Because only a few ounces of water would be expelled, it was not embarrassing to expel the water should someone come into the bathroom. Expelling two quarts of water was another matter. About the only time that I could use my two-quart enema syringe was when my roommate went home or away for the weekend. And even then, I would have to take the enema at a time the large common bathroom was not in heavy use.

Under the circumstances, I did not try to take seasonal enemas; I waited until I was home on vacation. About the only time I took either bag or bulb-type enemas was for acute spastic colon attacks, or when I had a cold. Use of heavy dosages of antibiotics was standard in those days, even for colds. Such antibiotic use would kill the good bacteria in my colon, which caused me to have a higher frequency of spastic attacks. The small-bulb enema brought me emergency relief. The small-volume, disposable type of enema units available on drugstore shelves today would have filled that emergency need for me, but of course they were not available in those days.

I was very active, and usually had daily bowel movements. During my first year of college, I took only one seasonal enema, and probably a half-dozen others at school. My other three seasonal enemas Fran gave me when I came home or during summer vacation. I did not have as much bowel comfort at school as when I was home, probably because of the stress of starting college, but I eventually found I could minimize stress by working hard and keeping ahead on my school work. In fact, my early successes at college were quite encouraging. My good start the first year set the trend for the rest of my college

experience. Mom, Fran, and I were exceptionally pleased with my bowel health, all things considered. We all feared disaster that first year because of the stress and change of diet. But soon I learned how important it was to manage stress. It became second nature for me. If I were careless managing stress or my diet, I would pay a high price.

I enjoyed living in the dorm. The food was surprisingly good. To this day, I would like to have a reunion with those I met that first year. I had a good roommate, and the guys on my floor were great. One was an English major and helped me a great deal with my compositions.

Doing the summer between my freshman and sophomore years, Mother arranged for me to have a full-scale medical exam at a well-known clinic. She wanted to be sure my bellyaches were for the same old reason of spastic colon. A doctor of internal medicine took a complete medical and lifestyle history. My heart, blood pressure, pulse, etc. were checked and found to be well within normal limits. My body was prodded, flexed and pushed from head to toe. The exam included extensive urinalysis and blood work-ups, including a six-hour blood sugar test. My kidneys were x-rayed after injecting radioactive materials into my blood. I swallowed barium

and had upper gastrointestinal x-rays. The procedure most relevant was the barium x-ray of my colon. This involved being taken down a hallway with several doors. A nurse escorted me through one door into a very small room, about 12'x 8'. Along the wall to my right was a long, padded, exam-type table. At the far end of the room was a toilet near the left wall, opposite the table. There was a locker on the left wall as well. The nurse abruptly said, "Please undress. You can leave your socks on. You can hang your clothing in the locker. Put the gown on that is lying on the table. I will be back soon to give you your enema."

This was really a surprise because no one had mentioned anything about my getting an enema. My sister had brought me to the clinic on this second day of tests. She either did not know or did not tell me what was scheduled. I undressed and jumped up on the exam table. Pretty soon the door opened, and the nurse hung a can on an inside door hook. It was a rather large enamel white can with a red hose curled around the hook. It had what appeared to be a large, grey, steel nozzle attached to the hose. The nozzle was about six inches long with a bulbular end with a circular spray head. The can was full of water, billowing at the top with white soapsuds. I could smell the

Castile soap, a smell I was familiar with. The nurse said nothing, and closed the door. I was obviously in a special enema room, probably one of several.

Pretty soon the nurse came in and said, "Please roll over on your left side. I want you to flex your legs, the top one more than the bottom one."

I heard the familiar snapping on of rubber gloves. Out of the corner of my eye I could see her lubricating her right index finger from a tube of K-Y jelly that she picked up from the small table.

She stepped over near me and said, "I need to check and lubricate your rectum; just relax." As she spoke, I could feel her spread my buttocks and start massaging my anus, not unlike Mom and Fran had done so many times before. Then she said, "Bear down like you are going to have a bowel movement." She pushed her finger deep into me and turned it a bit, then withdrew it.

She took down the nozzle and lubricated generously from the same tube of K-Y. "Okay, here we go," she said as she spread me open again, and pushed in the nozzle. I heard the familiar snap of the clamp. The water was warmer than I was used to, almost hot. I could feel the sting from the strong soapsuds solution. I realized why our

family doctor did not advise using sudsy water.

"The more you can take from this can, the fewer times we will have to do this," she said in a tone bordering on a command.

This was an extremely uncomfortable enema, like the one that I had when my appendix was removed.

I told her, "I'm going to bust; STOP, PLEASE!"

She replied, "You can do it." I begged her to stop as I cramped in pain. Finally she stopped the flow, and let me rest. I told her I could not take anymore. My belly was bulging. The nozzle delivered the enema at a speed I was not used to. I moaned in agony as she opened the clamp again.

"We only have a couple cups left," she said as she poured it into me.

I was writhing in agony as she pulled the nozzle out. She held a cloth tight against my anus. I was begging her to let me go, but she rolled me over on my back and pulled the gown up and gingerly massaged my abdomen in circular motions up the left side, across, and then down the right side.

She said, "I can see you have not had three quarts before." By now, I was oblivious to the passage of time.

She finally pulled a pan from under the cabinet and slid it under me and said, "You can go now."

I never dreamed so much could come out of a person at one time. After my belly went down a good bit she asked me to hold it, and pulled the bedpan from under me. She poured the contents of the bedpan into the toilet and sprayed it out with the special spray attachment. She then helped me onto the toilet, and left the room for me to finish. I was grateful, as I always preferred doing this in private, even at home.

After a while she came back into the room and asked if I was done. I said, "Yes." This was the second painful and traumatic enema I had received, ironically, again in a hospital setting.

She said, "Get back up on the table. I will be back in a few minutes."

She returned holding the largest enema bag I had ever seen. She hung it up on the same hook, and said, "Okay, over on your side." She started the whole routine again. The only difference was that she shoved a colon tube high up into me this time as she delivered this huge enema. Surprisingly, I took most of the bag comfortably. She then stopped the flow."

"You are doing fine, Mr. Wisner. Now turn over on your back. I need to massage your abdomen." Then she started the flow again.

The last part of the enema was extremely painful. I moaned and begged her to stop. Years later, I realized this was a four-quart bag.

"I am going to bust. Please stop."

"We are about done, Mr. Wisner."

I am sure they could hear me in the hallway. I hope no poor soul heard me before going into one of the other rooms. She withdrew the long colon tube, and slid the bedpan under me. The same routine again, but this time she said, "That is going to do it, Mr. Wisner. The flow is essentially clear. I know it's been a little rough, but you have done this in two rather than three or four steps."

I thought, *thank God*. I had received another harsh enema. No wonder so many people hated getting them.

She then escorted me out into the waiting room where several people sat around dressed in gowns, looking like me.

Pretty soon, another nurse called me. She escorted me into a darkened room where I came face to face with a man with a heavy apron, gloves, and a weird set of goggles

resting on his forehead. He looked to be from another planet. The nurse helped me onto the table in the center of the room. I looked up and saw a massive piece of equipment overhead that was obviously x-ray equipment. I could see an IV stand with a long plastic bag hanging from it full of a white-milky substance. This time, the nozzle draped around the IV stand looked like none I had ever seen. A latex line ran inside of two deflated balloons that were just a few inches apart. Attached to the line was what I came to know as a soft-plastic, barium enema nozzle. The nozzle was about six inches long with a large hole in the end with two holes in each side of its bulbular head.

"Okay Mr. Wisner, we are going to x-ray your colon, but first we have to start a barium enema." I saw the nurse squeeze huge amounts of lubricant over the nozzle apparatus. She told me to turn over. She spread my buttocks, and slid this into my rear. I could hear her pumping a bulb and could feel myself feeling full inside. Later, I learned she was pumping up a balloon inside me, then one outside of me. The balloons provided a tight seal. She then donned the same type of apron and gloves as the man's. I could hear her open the clamp. The man, obviously the radiologist, said very little, other than "start"

or "stop" the enema. Sometimes he would say, "more air," and I would feel movement inside of my colon, sometimes cramping me. The nurse pumped air into my colon when needed. He rolled me around as I heard the machine stop and start. At one point, the doctor elevated the table so that my feet were nearly straight up and my head down.

I can not explain why, but my penis became fully erect. There were no sexual feelings, however I tried repeatedly to cover my erection with my hand, but the radiologist kept pushing my hand aside. Apparently, my hand was getting in the way of the filming.

After quite a while, I heard air releasing, and the nurse pulling out all of the apparatus from my rear. The doctor said, "Good job, Mr. Wisner." The doctor and nurse helped me to step down from the table. I was shown where the toilet was and instructed to void as much of the barium solution as I could. I felt most of the barium leave my bowels quickly.

The report from my complete "executive physical," as it was called, was that everything looked fine, including my colon. I was nineteen years old, and after years of enemas my colon was pronounced to be in excellent shape.

I looked forward to going back to college, but I

preferred more privacy than dormitory living provided. I liked complete quiet for studying, a trait I was forced to give up in later years because most work places are not quiet. I preferred to sit down all alone in a comfortable chair and study. Part of me was a loner who enjoyed living in my own place under warm and snug conditions.

So during that summer, I looked around for a room out in town. After the first year, the university allowed students to live anywhere they wished. I found the perfect place. It was a traditional house near campus. It was an attic-type apartment. The stairs leading to the second floor were inside but private. A locked door at the bottom of the stairs led to the landlord's quarters. The apartment had a large bedroom, good size living room and a large bathroom with tub. The bedroom came furnished with a large bed, dresser and full mirror. The living room had a an ample sofa, tea table, and television. It was warm and snug-perfect for me, and was very private. If I took an enema, I could hang the bag to dry in the bathroom and did not have to worry about anyone's questions. I stayed there for the remainder of my college years. My landlord was a pleasant widow who was respectful of my privacy. After a few months she insisted that I call her Doris. From time to time, she invited me

down for a visit. She lived alone. She was very good company on those visits. Although she was an older woman, she was still quite attractive, and had aged gracefully.

Although Fran or Mom still gave me occasional enemas when I was home or in the summer, I was mainly giving them to myself. Because of my new found privacy, I gave myself three of my four seasonal ones during my second year of college. I was having fewer spastic-colon attacks. Counting colds and acute attacks, I probably gave myself about a half-dozen enemas during the first year in the apartment. I did have periods of discomfort, but I tried to limit my use of enemas as long as I had good bowel function and did not have acute attacks. However, I had not learned the value of periodic enemas for me between the seasonal ones, nor had I discovered all of the secrets for almost total bowel comfort. However, I was learning. In addition to becoming good at stress management, I intuitively discovered that certain foods, or combinations of foods, would cause a spastic attack. A good example was pancakes. How I loved pancakes, but as the old saying goes, "They did not love me."

For a long time I sensed that it was good for me to

masturbate after having an enema. During my second year of college I consciously realized the value of masturbating after each enema, if I was in the mood at all. Also, I had always known that being "a little horny" made enemas easier to take. On the other hand, being "too horny" was a detriment because I would get too tense, and could not relax. When I was extremely tense I masturbated before having the enema to become relaxed. So I deliberately planned, and would even wait a bit, if at all possible, to take an enema until I felt at least a slight need to masturbate. This planning was not difficult because I was masturbating most days of the week. Many times, the enema itself would give me the stimulus to masturbate because it provided extraordinary stimulation, and the prostate gland felt completely drained after ejaculation. Ejaculation, especially when draining the prostate fully, has always been a healthful activity for me, not to mention stress relieving, and pleasurable. I have read that there is no way to drain the prostate more completely than through intercourse. This may be true. Married men are said to be healthier than single men. I think they are healthier, sexually, for sure. I have read that after masturbation, the penis goes soft slowly, as compared to after intercourse.

However, I have found that my penis resolves (goes soft) almost as fast as after intercourse when I masturbate after having an enema. I have found it to be true, that it takes a lot longer for my penis to resolve after I masturbate without using enemas. In other words, I feel I get the best and most complete drains after sexual intercourse or after enema use. For me, the best of both worlds is intercourse after having an enema.

I dated regularly during the early part of college, and as in high school, many of my dates would tell me that they had never been with a more erotic date. Although I neither took a girl up to my apartment, nor had intercourse with any, I continued to masturbate after dates, even sometimes before. I was fortunate to find that many girls enjoyed hot petting sessions just as much as I did. Some wanted to be brought to orgasm by digital and oral means, just short of intercourse. Fortunately, some chose, and enjoyed immensely, seeing and feeling me in the throes of intense orgasm. They achieved this by pleasuring me by hand, or by performing oral sex. As fastidious as I was, I never seemed to mind the mess, nor did they. I enjoyed pleasing them orally, and tasting their juices. I love to hear a woman cry out from intense pleasure. Restraint from

intercourse may sound odd to many younger readers, but this was a time before the "pill", and the sexual revolution. Conception was to be avoided at all costs. The moral restraints were much greater then, for better or for worse. Even now, I think it depends upon the particular circumstances when it comes to premarital sex. It would be great if there were an easy answer, but I do not think there is an answer which fits all situations. In the early part of this century, boys and girls married soon after reaching puberty. Today, many men and women are interested in intercourse for many more years before they marry. More and more men and women never marry.

Today I wonder, why oh why, I did not find those many enemates early. I suppose it was good because I likely would have married too soon. I really wasn't emotionally ready for marriage. I met many whom I truly loved sexually, loved as persons, and was compatible with in every other way. In finding an enemate whom I loved, marriage would have been impossible to resist.

Another unique experience that I had in college was my first colonic irrigation. The only place that offered the service was in a large city over one hundred miles away. So when Doris needed to visit her doctor in the same city, I

offered to drive her. She had a genetic heart condition and needed a checkup. After her appointment her sister, Phyllis, was going to pick Doris up at the doctor's office. After their visit, I was to meet them later at the sister's house. This gave me the opportunity to make an appointment for a colonic irrigation. I would pick Doris up later in the afternoon after my colonic, and we would then head back to the university.

I arrived on time at the colon therapist's office, which was on the tenth floor of a tall downtown office building. I was nervous, to say the least. However, she did everything to make me feel comfortable. She asked me a lot of medical history-type questions first. She was very laid back and did not rush me. She then pointed to the bathroom and asked me to empty my bladder, which I did. She then showed me to the colonic irrigation room. She directed me where to hang my clothes. The room was long and narrow. There was an exam-type table along one wall. There was a huge glass tank full of water on a ledge. Connected to the tank was a hose. Attached to the hose was a very small, stainless- steel, bullet-shaped nozzle affair with a hole in the end. She pointed to a gown on the table for me to put on after I had undressed. I undressed, put the gown on, and

got up on the table.

Soon I heard a knock on the door, "Are you ready, Mr. Wisner?"

I nervously responded, "Yes."

"Mr. Wisner, please roll over on your left side. I need to give you a rectal exam before we start."

I heard her snap on a rubber glove. "Okay Mr. Wisner, bear down a little and we will check you out."

This therapist, like all to follow, had the talent for inserting a gloved finger, nozzle, or speculum with painless ease. It still never ceases to amaze me. I hardly felt her finger go in. Once it was in, she probed around, causing me no pain. Just before she withdrew her finger, she massaged my prostate, and then did what she called "stripping it."

"Did that feel good, Mr. Wisner"

I responded, almost breathlessly, "Oh my God, yes!"

"That's good, Mr. Wisner. You are fine in there."

To this day, I always benefited from a gentle prostate massage. It always makes me feel better and healthier. When that pure, clear prostatic fluid pours out my penis, I intuitively feel that any stale stuff left in there has been forced out. People who know how to massage and strip my

prostate can do this without causing pain, nearly making me ejaculate but not. I can tell when they do some good because I feel a slight burning in the urethral tract.

She then turned me on my back with my knees raised and feet flat. She inserted the small nozzle, and opened the clamp. The water started flowing into my colon. Amazingly, this small nozzle stayed in on its own. Looking back now, I have never had a colonic like this since. Most insert a speculum with a drain hose attached, and a water input hose fastened into the side of the speculum. There were no gauges or the like with this setup, just the water running in through this small bullet-shaped nozzle. When the colon got full enough, or under enough pressure, the contents of the colon would just flush out around the small nozzle naturally, and fall into a small trough that emptied into a pipe to the sewer.

This was a simple system, yet it worked amazingly well. There was slightly more odor because it was not a closed system. The therapist massaged my belly as we discussed my diet and other helpful things. She was quite interested in my spastic colon history. She noticed my appendectomy scar, and asked me about that. She refilled the glass container from time to time with various

temperatures of water, which was pleasant.

After many gallons of water going in and out for about an hour, she shut the water off, and slid the small nozzle out of my rectum.

"You did fine, Mr. Wisner. Now go in the bathroom and empty out any water that remains in your colon."

I went into the bathroom and let the small amount of water that remained in my bowel out. I did notice something that would be a common sight for me after colonic. In the area of my penis, my gown would be soaked with prostatic fluid. Years later, I asked a therapist about this. She told me that some men experience some sexual excitement, which causes the secretion. For others, it is just natural after the pressure and heat on the prostate. I think, for me, it is a combination. Sometimes I experience some sexual excitement during the process, but I have always known this. Therapists understand, and think nothing of it. During some colonic irrigations, my penis will become fully erect. At other times it will not become erect at all. Other times, my penis is like a flag going up and down. Sometimes my penis remains at half mast. It just depends upon my sexual state before the procedure.

When my penis is erect, it is obvious to the therapist.

Even when covered, the therapist may brush the head of my penis during massage, but neither of us gives it any thought. As a patient, I have become like the professional therapist. I know it is happening, but do not think about it in a sexual way. I do think, however, the secretion of prostatic fluid is good for me.

It takes several good and high enemas to do the job of the colonic irrigation. Even then, I do not think an enema is ever as thorough as the colonic cleansing.

The hydrotherapy was good for my body, and the hydro therapist good for my soul and spirit. I came down on the elevator feeling a little weak, even though she had given me some juice to drink. She advised me to have some yogurt or buttermilk to help restore the bacterial flora in my bowel. I felt wonderful the next day after a good night's sleep; in fact, I felt extra good for many days to follow.

My landlord's sister lived in the suburbs, in the same direction as the university. Phyllis insisted on feeding us supper before we started back. It was a good idea because I needed to rest. We all had a good time. Phyllis was a widow, too. We had a wonderful supper of roast beef, potatoes and vegetables cooked to perfection.

In the early evening, Doris and I headed back toward

the university. She asked me if I had a good time. I said, "Your sister is wonderful. Yes, I had a wonderful day."

She asked me, "I hope you did not have a hard time spending the day while I went to the doctor and visited with my sister?"

I said, "No, there has been something I have been wanting to do for a long time and I finally got it done." I explained to her that I went to a health care professional as well. I explained that I had a spastic colon condition all of my life, and I went to a specialist to try a treatment.

Much to my surprise she said, "Did you try a colonic irrigation?"

Astonished, I blushed a bit and said, "Why yes, how did you know about colonic irrigation?"

"My husband had a spastic colon problem and colonic irrigations helped him. It's okay, nothing to be ashamed of."

It turned out that her husband had gone to the same therapist as I did.

"Have you taken enemas for it, too?"

Blushing just a bit, I said, "Yes, many, since I was a child."

"My husband, too. I was pretty sure you took enemas."

"How would you know?"

"Do you remember when you asked me to go up into your living room and get the term paper to give to the friend that stopped by? I could not help but see the four-quart enema bag hanging in plain view in your bathroom. That is not a bag used by a beginner."

"Gosh, I forgot I left it out in the open."

We went on talking about most everything. We knew each other a lot better after that trip. I discovered I had much in common with her departed husband. Doris and I became close friends that day.

I drove up and parked the car in the street in front of her house. I thanked her for all the courtesy shown to me. I especially wanted her to know I appreciated living in her home. I told her how nice I thought her sister was.

She reached over and kissed me on the check and said, "You're welcome, Charlie."

Before we separated, she said, "Look Charlie, I am not a young woman. I have been through a lot, and know people pretty well. I think a lot of you, Charlie. Should you ever need any help with an enema, just let me know. Neither one of us should feel embarrassed if you need my assistance. It is something I know how to do. I know how

much easier it is to be given one than to do it yourself. Please do not hesitate to ask me for help."

I responded, "Thanks, there are times that I could use your help."

Over the last three semesters of school, I had a helper with enemas. I even took a few just for the pleasure to share intimacy with Doris. I explained how my mother and Fran had given them to me. Doris did not need much instruction as to technique, or as to loving and caring.

Because of her experience with her husband, she was able to pass on some things she had learned from his experience. One thing she learned about her husband was that if she gave him a periodic enema series, he would rarely have an acute spastic-colon attack. After considerable trial and error with her giving me enemas, we discovered that if I took a monthly series that I would rarely have an acute attack, and I found great comfort between enemas, rather than growing discomfort until the next attack.

We also learned of the best sequence and positioning for me. The first one was given on the left side in bed, and the second in the knee-chest position on the bathroom floor. The third enema was given on my back on the bed with

several pillows under my pelvis. It turned out that I had serendipitosly met an expert enema giver who was able to pass on some specific knowledge learned from her experience with her husband. As luck would have it, those lessons were applicable to me. I was able to assist her also a couple of times.

I felt this intimate and personal contact was helping me and Doris in more ways than one. She was very professional in helping me, but as time went by I noticed her face grimace as she administered my enema on my back. I was in position to see her face clearly. By the time she had given me several on my back, formalities were dropped. For enemas, I usually wore a nightshirt over briefs. For the enema I would pull down my briefs just enough to expose my butt. But it was more convenient and easier just to strip them off, rather than pull them halfway down. Once I was on top of the pillows, with my feet flat near the edge of the bed, my head sloping back toward the center of the bed, I would pull up my nightshirt. My genital area would be fully exposed. Doris would sit on a chair between my parted legs to give the enema. I would pull my legs up and Doris would first lubricate my rectum. I noticed that each time she was going deeper; finally, she

was touching my prostate. I'm sure she noticed my low groans and wriggles of pleasure. She started losing her breath when she grimaced. She was a woman in the throes of orgasm. After lubricating, should would insert the nozzle, and I would drop my feet flat again, and the enema would be given.

One day, a few months before I was to be graduated, I called her to ask if she had time to give me an enema series. I had taken more enemas than I needed. In my mind I wished for something more, but would never ask for it.

"Of course, Charlie, I always have time for you."

After the first two enemas my bowel was clean. I positioned myself on my back for the third enema as usual. With my pelvis raised high upon four pillows, I asked her, "Doris, will you massage my prostate? It feels like I need it." I believed it did because I had been feeling some irritation after ejaculation. I had been masturbating frequently recently, probably to excess. To this day, I feel that masturbation is harmless, but if done too frequently my prostate tires and does not completely drain its contents. I theorize that remnants left deep in the prostate become stale and cause irritation. Even slight irritation causes me to masturbate even more to get rid of the irritation, setting up

a cycle. This theory may also be partially based upon some readings sometime in the past.

She replied, "My husband also needed his prostate massaged from time to time. Sure Charlie, whatever you want. I always enjoyed doing it for him."

I could see a smile on her face, even a gleam in her eye of anticipation.

After several delightful minutes, I gasped and blurted out, "Oh Doris, please suck my penis while you are massaging my prostate. Do you mind?" I asked without thinking. But with the request came an intuitive assurance that I was safe asking Doris to do this. I knew I could trust her, even if she refused. I had bonded to Doris, just as I had with my own mother and Fran, but in an additional way.

With her finger still pushing deep within me, she said, "Whatever you want, my young man."

She bent down and put her parted lips over the head of my penis and began sucking, obviously to both of our enjoyment. Then, I felt that now familiar intense surge rolling through my genitals. I then erupted, and could feel my juices spattering inside her warm and wet mouth with each throb of my penis. She swallowed hard, and then looked at me in my eyes, and said, "I love you, Charlie, for

what you have done for me. I never dreamed that I would again experience such youthful things. I know I can trust you to be discreet."

I replied, "You can trust me forever, Doris, my love."

She kissed me with her wide mouth. This was one of the most erotic moments of my life.

I looked into her large brown eyes and asked, "After my enema, will you sleep with me?"

She said, "Yes, Charlie, I would like that. I would like that very much."

After my final enema, I bathed and then we lay together, embraced and kissed.

I asked her, "Doris, teach me."

"I will, my tender love," she replied.

Teach me, she did. We would spend many weekends and week nights together in this sweet, but discreet tryst. No one ever knew what went on in that house, but it was good and right. I loved this woman who was almost three times my age. It was obvious she loved me. She was a mixture of mother, friend, and lover. We loved each other for all the right reasons, while at the same time knowing our love was limited by circumstances, place, and time. I loved to hold her naked body next to mine for hours at a

time.

This was a grand opportunity for the two of us, two people who loved each other, knowing it was safe and no harm could come of it. I was a virgin who needed training, and she was an older woman with the experience and desire for the opportunity. It was an unusual linking of two people, but it was hot and wonderful. It was dear in every way. It would be hard to explain to the rest of a disapproving society, but it was clean and pure to us.

The first time Doris said, "I love you, Charlie," and then kissed me on the mouth, my mind flashed back to when Fran had first kissed me on the mouth and said, "I love you, Charlie." I now wondered if, deep down, Fran felt the same way about me as Doris did, and if she had desired more from me. But when that first happened I was still a child, and Fran would never have taken advantage of me. She was my mother's best friend, not to mention a professional nurse. Plus, my mother had entrusted me to her care. Yet, after that I wondered if Fran had ever dreamed of more. Had she struggled with her own desires? I know I had.

I soon was graduated from college. Doris, a mixture of third mother, friend and lover, attended my graduation

along with my mother and dad, Fran and her husband, Joe.

I had been in the Reserve Officers Training Corps throughout college, ROTC, and not only earned a B.S. degree, but also was graduated as a second lieutenant. I would soon be off to the army. Everyone medically fit served in those days, and I chose to go as an officer.

Before going into the army I stopped in for a day's visit with Doris. I can still remember crying in her arms. As I left town, I could not stop crying. Only the very busy days ahead could stop my tears.

I returned every time I could to my university town and my home away from home to be with my beloved Doris. It would be years before I would marry. I just could never forget Doris. She was my first love. My heart and soul burned for her.

Doris was always glad to see me, and I to see her. In between, we spent long hours on the phone keeping each other up to date. I loved to be with her, and to sleep with her when I could. We enjoyed late-night breakfasts at restaurants that gave us time out of the house. Everyone who saw us together no doubt figured we were just very good friends, similar to mother and son. She would come and visit me on occasion, wherever I was stationed

stateside. We would renew our passion for each other. We had great fun fooling people because of our age difference. Probably no one suspected that we were lovers. Most young people do not realize that passionate love and sex can go on into our senior years. Love never has to end just because of age. Doris taught me that.

I had lucked out because the enema had brought me good fortune again. The enema had opened the door of intimacy with my first love. The love between me and Doris was wonderful, but ended abruptly when I lost her only two years later due to a heart attack. As beautiful as she was, she could not overcome a genetic heart problem.

People probably wondered why I always wept at the mention of her name. I always had a way of remembering her. With the change of seasons, fresh flowers appeared on her grave. I was lost without her. She could never be replaced, of course. Would I ever find another enemate to sparkle my life?

Soldier Boy

I lived virtually unaffected by two wars, WWII and The Korean War, but hardly any person was untouched by the long Vietnam War. As the war raged in Vietnam, discontent spilled upon the streets of America. I sometimes wondered which field of battle was worse. The war on the streets shared one ingredient with the one abroad-heartbreak.

I stayed in the army for several years. As a young officer, my first two years included lots of training and preparation. Vietnam was not going full tilt yet, but the war would accelerate, as would dissatisfaction at home with our involvement in Vietnam. I was stateside the first two years, which helped me to keep in contact with Doris.

Although age differences should have sent me on my way, I just could not get over her. Only her death ended the relationship. Doris would always be part of my soul. I suppose no one ever totally gets over a first love, even if it was "puppy love," but our love was more mature than that. Yes, she helped me to grow sexually, but "her talks" provided independent confirmation of my earlier ones with my mother and Fran. My responsibilities as a man toward

women is one example. I will always love Doris, God rest her soul.

I rarely got home during my military years. Without Mom, Fran, or Doris, enemas were self-administered, but only when beyond necessity. Now enemas lacked the love component that I had always been blessed with. During my life, almost all of my enemas were initiated for health reasons, but after her death I ignored my health. The loves in my life were no longer present to counteract the shocking events around me. I started living a cycle of acute spastic-colon attacks, then enemas, but only after experiencing deep pain. I ignored good health practices that I had discovered over the years, such as eating the right combination of foods and avoiding hard liquor. I would overeat, not exercise, and stress myself, not getting adequate rest. I stopped taking prevention enemas. I no longer felt good. Instead, my belly was uncomfortable and sore most of the time. I was not into any preventive health care. I was living in a tragic world and I lived a " just get by life." After Doris died, I could only see a world gone crazy. She was not there to help me to appreciate life. I even began to binge drink, which always ended with harsh vomiting, something I hated.

Finally, I decided to get out of the army. I was stationed stateside, just "killing time" before I mustered out, but it would be several months yet. That is when I met Jenny.

Jenny was a small woman compared to Doris, who was 5'8". Jenny was only 5'2", and just over one hundred pounds. Although she was twenty-four years old, she looked like an innocent school girl of sixteen. She had a bright and clean complexion, and a wholesome countenance that revealed her inner soul. Besides being of slight build, she was beautifully shaped, with light-brown hair and deep-blue eyes. Her long hair tumbled down her back in wavelets to below the belt of her jeans. I eventually discovered how beautiful and delicate her small breasts were, with the various shades of her nipples to highlight them.

Doris had been buxom compare to petit Jenny, but Jenny was pleasing to look at with her small, almost child-size ass, and tapered legs. When the light would passed between her legs it revealed her most erotic part, that part that designated her from birth to be a "split tail." Her pouted mound told all that she was now a woman who possessed the most beautiful flower of all as it lay in full bloom between her exquisite legs. Much later, she would

occasionally want me to trim her soft bush down to her butter-soft mound, allowing her vaginal opening to be seen as it cut through the dramatic arch of her pubic bone. Then the scant pubic hair would slowly grow back to its natural state.

Obviously, my initial attraction to her was physical. I can not explain the chemistry of sexual attraction, but it is strong, like a magnet. I had never been attracted to such a small woman before.

She was working as a hostess in the Officers Club and attending a local college, studying to become a teacher. Unlike myself, she had little free time, but I asked her out on a date the first night I spied her, something unusual for my reserved personality.

It was a traditional date. We went out to dinner and then to a movie. Her family lived in the same town, but she had her own apartment near the army post. She invited me to her place because it was a private place to be together. This gesture was not an invitation to have intercourse. I could not take her to my place, the Bachelor Officers Quarters.

Within a few dates we were passionately making out, but she was not about to jump into bed, which I would have

preferred. And even when we eventually made it over to her bed, the sexual boundary was giving each other orgasms digitally or orally. I asked her repeatedly to let me put a rubber on to "do it," but she refused to go all the way, even as hot as she was. We would be drenched with sweat, naked, and still she held out. Like most girls of the era, she had a paralyzing fear of getting pregnant. With her, getting pregnant before marriage would be the "mother" of all disgraces, even at twenty-four. Rubbers were only ninety-percent safe, and ten-percent failure was too great of a risk for her. After all the training given to me by mom, Fran and Doris, I could not fault her. There was not wide spread use of the "pill" to fuel the sexual revolution, which was just getting underway. Besides, she was born of my generation, rather than of the young and more liberal one.

I went out with Jenny only a short time before I did discovered that she was part of the newer generation in one respect. She was into health. She was not a "flower child," but was quite concerned about our environment and personal health care. She was an early one into drinking filtered water, and stood up vigorously for clean air and water. I went to several rallies with her that were benign efforts to speak to the politicians about environmental

concerns.

It was obvious to both of us that there was more to our relationship than mere physical attraction. We truly liked one another, and we respected each other.

Part of Jenny's health beliefs included eating a healthful diet. Because I had an acute spastic-colon attack one night, I confessed my lifelong problem. From that point on she was determined to get me into a healthful lifestyle, including diet. Because of her, I discovered the importance of eating enough fiber. Like many Americans, I was fiber deficient. She knew about spastic colon because she had read about it. She said it was now called Irritable Bowel Syndrome, IBS. She had read where many IBS sufferers benefit by ingesting adequate fiber. Once I ingested the recommended amount of daily fiber, my colon condition improved. Although increased fiber content was contraindicated for many IBS sufferers, I was in the lucky group that benefited from it. She also introduced me to drinking plenty of pure water daily, another advancement. In general, Jenny got me back into taking care of myself.

I began to be conscious again of stress management and staying away from foods I was allergic to. I began to feel much better. Jenny also taught me not to overeat at one

sitting. I gave up drinking booze. I was not very good at drinking anyway.

Jenny was so into health that I felt comfortable telling her that I had taken enemas since childhood. To my surprise, she beamed when I told her of this, and said, "Really, I think that is good for you. My mom gave me enemas until I was fourteen. After that, she and I went to a colon therapist regularly. It was a mother-daughter thing with us. I don't take an enema very often, but I continued the colonic irrigations regularly. Mother and I still go together sometimes. Mother believed in the health value of colonics. I believe that colonic irrigations have a lot to do with my good health. I believe, like the ancient Egyptians, that my good complexion is due to regular cleanses. You know, I never had adolescent acne. Have you ever had a colonic irrigation?"

"Why yes, I have. My first one was several years ago while in college. I went back a second time, but the therapist was a long way from the university." She asked me to describe the procedure.

She responded, "That's okay, Charlie, but she used very old equipment and the old gravity method. Up-to-date therapists today use better equipment and methods."

She described in detail the colonic irrigation equipment of the day, and how her therapist gave her a colonic.

"Charlie, I could make an appointment for both of us to get one, if you like."

I responded, " Jenny, I would appreciate that. With you along I would feel more comfortable. It is still hard to go the first time to a stranger for such an intimate thing."

She replied, "Don't worry, you'll be fine. My therapist is really nice."

The time for the appointment arrived. Jenny had made arrangements for her therapists to give me my colonic, and one of the partner therapists to give hers. This would allow us to finish about the same time.

We were called into separate rooms. Jenny's therapist was a kind and loving person, the type of person I was so used to.

After introducing herself she said, "Mr. Wisner, each of our colonic rooms have private bathrooms." Pointing, she said, "Please go into that one just off my office and empty your bladder." Pointing again, she said, "After you are done, go into the colonic room. Take off all of your clothes, and put on the hospital gown that is lying on the table. Sit on the table and I will be in soon."

I emptied my bladder and went into the colonic room, undressed, and then put on the gown and stepped up on the table that was similar to others I had seen. There was a disposable absorbent pad on the table. There was a square machine inset into the wall that had gauges in it and dials on it. There was a large rubber hose, about an inch in diameter lying on a small table along the opposite wall. Also on the small table was a gun-type device made of stainless steel. I guessed that was what she was going to insert into my rectum. It looked rather large. Attached to the machine was another hose that was about the size of an enema hose. Both of these hoses were a tan color and made of a gummy natural rubber.

The therapist gave me plenty of time to get ready, then knocked on the door.

"Ready?" she called.

I replied, "Yes."

She sat on a chair next to the table where I was sitting, and we began to talk. She asked many questions about my health, diet, lifestyle, etc.

"Okay Mr. Wisner, I now want to feel your abdomen, so lie down on your back."

She prodded and pushed until she was satisfied with my

condition.

"Now lie on your left side. We are going to examine your rectum."

I heard her snap rubber gloves on.

"O.K. now, Mr. Wisner, we are going to take a look. This will not hurt. You have had this done before. I will be very gentle."

I could barely feel her finger enter me. I could tell she was taking a good feel around.

As she touched my prostate she asked, "Did that hurt?"

I replied, "No."

As she withdrew her finger she said, "You look fine. Continue lying on your side. Pull your top leg up more toward your chest. I am going to put this speculum into your rectum now. It won't hurt."

I could feel her slide in the rather large stainless-steel piece that looked like a gun. It did not hurt. After it was inside me, I could feel her clamping the large rubber hose to the external end of the speculum.

"Mr. Wisner, this is the hose you will expel into. It goes from you into a pipe under the table. That pipe is a drain into the sewer. I'm attaching the smaller hose from the machine into the side of the external part of the

speculum. This is the water input hose. I can control the temperature and the pressure of the water going into your colon with valves and monitoring gauges. When there is enough water inside of you, or the water reaches a certain pressure, I will then turn a valve and stop the inflow of water. Next, I open the valve into the drain hose and empty you. This ebb and flow of water in and out of your colon will clean you out thoroughly and efficiently all the way around to the cecum. The cecum area is generally at the end of the small intestine and at the beginning of the large bowel, or the colon. We will eventually work all the way up your descending colon on your left side, then across the top, your transverse colon, then down the right side of your body, the ascending colon. We will alternate the pressure and temperature of the water, which will exercise and tone your colon in addition to cleansing it. It takes several enemas to do the job of the colonic irrigation. With the enema you can not vary the temperature, or even the pressure precisely. Now go over on your back. I prefer you to keep your legs raised with your feet flat. However, if you get tired you can lie with your legs down a while. We will put several gallons in and out of you. It will take forty-five minutes to an hour. I will be massaging your belly

throughout a good portion of this procedure. By the way, I am an R.N., a massage therapist, and a trained and licensed colonic therapist."

One thing I had noted was how clean her place was, and I told her how much I appreciated it.

She then went on. "Mr. Wisner, from your history, you have had many enemas. You are used to this type of intimate procedure. I prefer to pull your gown up to message a bare belly. I like to massage directly on the skin so I can feel your insides better. If exposing your private parts makes you uncomfortable, I will cover them. I do not want to embarrass you in any way."

With a sense of trust, I told her, "No, that is okay. You should know that I have a history of erecting with enemas and my prostatic fluid seeps out my penis. It is just natural with me. I don't always get an erection, but almost always seep fluid. Nothing is meant by it."

She replied, "No, that is just normal. I pay no attention to that. It just makes my job a lot easier if I do not have to work around and through towels and gowns. If you were not so experienced, I would not ask until you had several colonics and were more confident. If you were still anxious, I would not ask then. Most patients are

comfortable with me, knowing I am a nurse. Thank you; now we will start."

She opened the inflow of water and I could feel warmth enter me. She pulled up my gown and started to massage my belly, starting on the left side. This day I did not get an erection, but did seep prostatic fluid. The colonic was very pleasant. She was outstanding at this work. I could feel her knead my belly. I can understand why she preferred not to cover me. It was as if she could feel everything in my abdomen. Her kneading began just above the pubic hair line, and she worked her way up my left side, then eventually all of the way around. There was no doubt she was giving me a through cleansing. At other times I could feel cool water enter me, then warm water again.

"Mr. Wisner, we are done."

With those words, she eased out the speculum, and helped me up. She had me step on a small step stool down onto the floor. She directed me back to the bathroom to empty any water that could be left in my colon. There was not much.

After I came out of the bathroom and dressed, she gave me a glass of juice. She assured me that the hoses and speculum would be sterilized before use on others, just as

she had done before I came in. She had several spare sets, and told me how important sterilization was to prevent any cross contamination in patients. This assurance made me feel confident, once more, in her professionalism.

(These days, colon therapists usually use disposable plastic hoses and speculum. A plastic speculum does not go in quite as easily as a stainless steel one, but cross-contamination problems are eliminated because each unit is disposable. Assuming one does not have to travel very far, the only disadvantage to a colonic is its cost. Then it was only $25 for a session. I pay $50.00 today. In other parts of the country they can be much more expensive, even $100.)

The therapist wanted to give me a series of colonics. She said that it was not critical, but better health results could be achieved from an initial series. I felt good about her methods and modern colonics, so I enthusiastically agreed and set my next appointment.

I thanked her. She patted me on the shoulder and said, "You did fine, Mr. Wisner. By the way, call me Susan."

"Okay Susan. We're going to be seeing a lot of each other, so call me Charlie."

She smiled and replied, "Okay, Charlie it is."

Jenny met me in the lobby. She was waiting for me. I

looked upon her radiant face, now sure that it was more than genetics that gave her that healthy glow on her face.

On the way to her apartment she asked how I felt. I said, "A little weak, but great!"

She then said, "After a colonic, I like to go home and take a warm shower, get under the covers, and rest. We have bathed our insides; now let's go home and bath our outsides. Would you like to take a shower with me? It would be nice to have someone wash my back."

"I would like that, Jenny."

Jenny went on, "Then let's get under the covers all nice and clean, and NAKED!"

I replied, "Yes, that would be great!"

I looked forward to melding our bodies together. We got home, got into the shower together, washed each other's back, dried off, and crawled into bed.

We embraced and hugged as usual. We fell asleep for some time. When we awakened, I touched her lovely small breasts. I was quite horny. I noticed Jenny was unusually quiet and contemplative.

"What is it, Jenny?" I asked.

"Charlie, I need to talk with you about something. This is difficult for me, but I need to get it in the open. When

you take an enema and insert the nozzle, or the colon therapists insert a speculum, does it feel good? I mean real good?"

"Yes Jenny, it does. It has since I can remember."

"Charlie, I'm anal erotic. It feels very good to me. You know how putting your finger around my clitoris makes me feel so good. I'm a lot that way anally. Does that make any difference in how you feel about me? That's just the way I am."

"Jenny, it doesn't make any difference because I am also anal erotic. I think it's wonderful that we are compatible in this way, and I'm thrilled that you think it's important enough to tell me. Now we know that we have something else in common. We have an extra dimension of sexuality. I think most people are anal erotic, but it has not been awakened in them. I think we are both blessed. I appreciate your honesty. I've been trying to get around to telling you the same thing. If we are to have a long-term relationship, it's important for us to know these things. Sharing anal eroticism and colonic irrigations can strengthen our relationship.

"Charlie, I know you want me. I have gone as far as I can go vaginally. But there is more I can give if you want

to experiment. I have never had a penis in my rear, but I crave yours, Charlie. I want you to have anal intercourse with me. I'm like you, fastidious, but after a colonic I am clean down there. I want you, Charlie. I need you bad, Charlie. I want all of you, please."

"Do you think it will hurt, Jenny?"

"Charlie, may I be honest with you?"

"Of course, Jenny."

"Ever since I have been getting colonics, starting at age fourteen, I have come home and penetrated myself with my fingers, smooth objects, and for several years now, a large vibrator. Since puberty, I have been able to bring myself to orgasm anally, as well as by rubbing my clit."

"How should we go about it the first time, Jenny?"

"Make love to me like you always do. But it will be very helpful for us if you prepare my anus just before you enter me. It will stretch a great deal by use of your fingers. First, insert one finger, then more. Then I want you to insert the large vibrator I have, and turn it on, and work it in and out a bit. Then reinsert your fingers and stretch me even more. You will be amazed. Use a lot of Vaseline. Charlie, I will like it, believe me. I have fantasized about getting it in several different ways and positions, but the

first time I would like to kneel down on the edge of the bed with my butt facing out. You are just about the right height to give it to me as you stand. O.K.?"

"Jenny, I have those same erotic feelings. You have just the right man. I think we'll will have great fun."

Jenny set the jar of Vaseline and vibrator on the nightstand, and then we started to make love. We embraced and kissed. We both loved to feel each other's skin against our own. I loved her long hair that flowed down her back. She was so small, but exotic. Our kissing became ever more impassioned. I slid my wet tongue down to her small, but turgid breast. First, I encircled each nipple with my tongue, then suckled them gently. I began to feel her breathing heavily and moaning softly.

I traced her belly with my tongue down to her belly button, while gently taking the palm of my right hand and cupping her mound. I raised briefly to view her pubic area. She was such a small thing. Her tapered legs connected to her butt, which was no larger than a child's. She was so perfect and beautifully formed. She had legs and butt of the design and grace of the bottom half of a frog.

I was always amazed how small women seemed to be almost all pussy between their legs. I wondered if women

her and touched her anus with the head.

"I'm there, Jenny, back up on me. Be careful, I do not want to hurt you."

She was so little, and I was afraid that in her heat she would hurt herself when she impaled herself upon my member, which now looked like a slightly bent rod.

Much to my surprise, she wriggled just a moment, and quickly took my swollen penis in to its hilt. I begin to move in a gentle rhythm with her. She felt tight on my shaft. We were both now in the throes of ecstasy. I was still amazed how she could accomplish this feat, and with such ease. Her anal opening was flexible, even loose at times.

I could not help but powerfully thrust upon her as my penis swelled even more. I could feel deep within my pelvis the early spasms of orgasm. I reached around and massaged her drenched clit. She had one orgasm after another. I was in fear she would pass out from the intense pleasure.

With each orgasm she clamped down tighter on my shaft. My ejaculation began, but was held back by her growing tightness. I was now in extreme erotic pain without the needed relief. I was screaming in agony as I

could not ejaculate. Then she relaxed just a moment. I exploded. I filled her innards with my warm juices, which caused her an overwhelming orgasm that squeezed me dry.

We both fell forward onto the bed, then gently over on our left sides. I was unable to disengage my swollen penis from her. We lay there side by side. She had one last orgasm. She shuddered to a stop. Finally, my penis started to resolve. She moaned softly as it shrank and withdrew on its own.

She rolled over and kissed and kissed me.

"Charlie, you are everything I ever dreamed of. Don't ever leave me. Thank you, thank you, thank you."

I felt the same, and as I kissed her, I told her that I loved her.

I picked her small sensuous, body up and placed her gently in the center of the bed. I lay down next to her. We fell asleep in exhaustion. She would not let me have vaginal intercourse with her, but she gave me everything else she could.

We awakened and lay there for hours, holding and kissing each other, enjoying the afterglow. By morning, we had repeated this joy twice again, more subdued than the first time, yet sweeter. Although still a virgin, she was full

of my warm sperm. I never dreamed two people could enjoy anal intercourse as much as we. It was if we had saved up a whole lifetime of yearning for this night. We could have twice the joy, the "back door," and in the near future, the "front door" sex. What a blessing for us.

We spent most of the weekend in each other's arms. We knew that we were meant for each other. There was no doubt about our future together. The die was cast.

Enemates Forever

Jenny and I fell deeper and deeper in love. Two people could not be happier with each other. I mustered out of the army, took a temporary job locally, and moved into a small apartment in the same building as Jenny's. We were all but living together. We continued the routine of going for a monthly colonic irrigation together. We would give each other an enema if the other were ill. We discovered if we felt a cold coming on we could usually head it off by a timely enema, drinking fruit juices, taking a couple of aspirin and getting plenty of bed rest. If I felt the early warnings of an IBS attack Jenny gave me the quick help I needed.

As time passed our relationship grew rather than diminished. We were two truly compatible people. As Christmastime neared, I felt the romantic urge to ask Jenny to marry me. Her answer was an enthusiastic yes. She accepted with an outpouring of hugs and kisses. This was a very special Christmas for both of us. Jenny was scheduled to finish school in May, so June was a perfect time for this new elementary teacher to wed.

The engagement period provided more proof that we

were compatible on all important fronts, including liking and respecting each other's parents and friends. We both understood the important role our families would play in a marriage.

Remarkably, it would be both families' belief in the use of enemas and colonic irrigation that provided the initial common ground to bond both sets of parents together. The families knew of the other's belief even before they met. Jenny told her mother and father about my lifelong IBS problem and my use of enemas. She explained that I was going to her colon therapist. They also knew Jenny had given me a couple of emergency enemas. Her family was also aware of my family's health and religious beliefs regarding enema use. Jenny was also aware that Fran was like a second mother to me.

In turn, I was pleased to tell my family about Jenny's family's beliefs regarding health and the role the colonic therapy played in their lives. Although Jenny's family emphasized the colonic irrigation more, it was still the same general belief. My family was probably as comfortable with the home enema therapy as Mom and Fran were nurses. I was pleased to tell Mother and Fran how much help Jenny had been to me. My mother and Fran

took great comfort in knowing "their boy" was being well cared for, not only by enemas and colonic irrigations, but by Jenny's positive influence regarding my health, especially as they realized that I had not been taking care of himself since Doris's death.

It was wonderful how both families got along so well. I am still in wonder how the intimate nature of enema use can bring people together, and so quickly. It is a common ground to have with others. I have found this to be true in my many hours of discussion in recent years with those of similar beliefs, as discovered in chats on the Internet.

Prior to marriage, we continued our monthly colonic irrigation, but found ourselves giving each other enemas weekly, as much for pleasure as for health reasons. This afforded us the opportunity to get to know each other as enemates, and for at least weekly anal intercourse. I learned that it was patience, lubrication, and preparation that made anal intercourse so easy. Jenny and I were not into the practice of "fisting," but Jenny could painlessly take all of my large fingers up to my knuckles. In our anal play it was not long before my anus stretched enough to take almost all of Jenny's small fist. A weekly enema did not seem to diminish our bowel functions, but we both agreed that

weekly may be too often in the long run.

This was a time of learning about every form of substitute sex, something both of us were used to all of premarital lives, except for my brief time with Doris. I loved to spread Jenny's tiny tapered frog legs and give her cunnilingus, something she would enjoy immensely. She had a massive pubic area, which was more pronounced by a generous pubic arch.

I loved for her to please me orally. She could play me like an instrument. A special joy was for her to suck me to climax as she massaged my prostate, something Doris had introduced me to, and I, in turn, taught Jenny.

We were eagerly looking forward to vaginal intercourse after marriage. When we were married, the delayed anticipation made vaginal sex even more exciting. We become vaginal intercourse devotees, even more so than our earlier anal sex.

Jenny wanted to continue her career as an elementary school teacher for a time, but birth control would not be a top priority after marriage because we wanted children. This period prior to marriage would never be forgotten, even though it was without vaginal intercourse. It was a period of unforgettable and pleasurable enemas, colonic

irrigations, as well as oral and anal sex.

The wedding was a conservative, but grand affair. We lovebirds retreated to the mountains of eastern Colorado for our honeymoon.

Yes, we had enjoyed heavy petting, enemas, colonic irrigations, and anal sex prior to marriage, but regular vaginal intercourse, with all of its variations, opened up a whole new world, especially for the virginal Jenny. She was like a child in a sexual candy store. And, oh how I was infatuated with this small, but erotic woman, an infatuation that would continue throughout our marriage. Our honest communication would forever enrich our marriage.

The first time Jenny and I had frontal intercourse, I tried to digitally prepare her vagina, but it hurt too much. She was a true virgin, and her vault was still mostly covered with the hymen. She experienced minimal pain the first few times because I would get her very excited by clitoral stimulation, then gently move ahead after she was soaked with desire. It took a while before her vagina would loosen as her rectum had. She had spent many years in anal play. As she told me, she enjoyed it for years after every colonic she had since the age of fourteen. Soon, Jenny's vagina *introitus* loosened to fit me.

My penis turned out to be just the right length for her. If my penis were much longer it would have struck her cervix. As it was, if I thrust too hard and deep I would strike it causing her pain, so I'm glad not to be well endowed. Jenny's orgasms are powerful, and her vaginal muscle grips my penis with all the strength that I can tolerate. We consummated our marriage on our wedding night, then too many times to count over the years. We continued to enjoy occasional anal sex as a variant, but Jenny was now free to express herself in the way most women crave most, to fill her vagina with life-giving semen.

We loved the east slope of the Rocky Mountains north of Denver, and decided to move there. I found a good position in a bank, and Jenny turned out to be the kind of dedicated fourth-grade teacher every elementary school wanted to hire. Our marriage seemed made in heaven. Both of our families were welcome to visit us as often as they wished, and vice versa. We both enjoyed having them visit. Fran was never forgotten, and Jenny treated her like the second mother that she was. As it turned out, I was considered to be the child Fran could never have.

Time passed on, both of our careers progressed well,

and we enjoyed our work.

The monthly colonic irrigation routine in our lives was replaced with a monthly enema series because we liked the greater intimacy of giving each other enemas. Our first enema of the series is given to each other on the left side, the second in the knee-chest position. The third, and last in the series, is given on our back, feet set flat near the edge of the bed, butt raised with pillows, and head sloping back toward the middle. Our legs are spread at the knees for the ease of administration by the other. By helping each other in this way, the work is left to the giver, and the receiver can relax. This leaves the receiver's hands free to massage the belly. We achieve total penetration of the pure water we use by the third in the series. It is quite easy to hear the water sloshing around on the lower right of the ascending colon. We have found these positions to be quite efficient, not to mention, sexually exciting.

We still have occasional anal intercourse after an enema series, but we usually reserve that for after our two-a-year colonic irrigation. Jenny and I enjoy loving each other under any circumstances, but to this day, we find sexual intercourse to be a heightened experience after the sexual organs have been stimulated by an enema or colonic

irrigation. Jenny always massages my prostate just before the third enema in the series, much to my delight. I have been told that as long as my prostate is healthy, there is no harm if this if done with reasonable care. I would still go to a urologist if I had a prostate problem, and you can be sure Jenny does not wear long nails; Jenny has never thought giving up long nails to be a sacrifice. The enema series is not as thorough or toning as the colonic, but we hate to miss the intense intimacy we share by giving each other enemas.

With the monthly enema series, healthful diet, adequate fiber and water, not overeating at one setting, avoiding foods to which I'm allergic, and stress control, I have lived an almost normal life. Acute attacks of IBS have been almost eliminated. Jenny also insists on regular exercise of one form or another.

During our marriage one or the other of us has been sick and has taken enemas several days in a row, but it is rare that we are sick and space them any closer than within 7-10 days. Our standard use has been monthly. The personal test for us has been, Does the enema or colonic therapy improve bowel function, not diminish, or make it dependent? We have learned much about ourselves. Most

people are not willing to apply that much concentration to the subject. We generally consider daily bowel movements as normal for us, unassisted by enemas or laxatives. We do not want to be overly concerned with bowel function, but Jenny and I feel that it is unhealthful for us to accept poor function. We just can not buy into what some doctors and books say these days; i.e., whatever is normal for you is okay, even if it is several days between bowel movements. Our colon muscles are strong enough that we usually have a bowel movement the day after an enema or colonic.

The monthly enema series (or colonic therapy) as part of my health regimen pays great dividends in bringing me comfort from IBS. I do not fully understand why. It could be the exercising and stretching of the colon, cleansing it, or the placement of warm soothing water, or a combination of these or other factors. I am also quite aware of eating foods to assist in replacing the bowel flora which enemas and colonic can deplete.

We have told a few of our non-enema-taking friends about our enema practice, and some of their responses are similar to: You poor things, that you have to do that; or, Ugh-nasty. We have never thought of the enema or colonic irrigation as something dirty. We think of them as

cleansing. The worst one can say about the enema is that one experiences what everyone else does, a bowel movement.

When we have told a few friends that they were even pleasant when properly given, they have looked at us in disbelief. Jenny's answer to them has always been, Have you not noticed the smile on an infant's face after he or she empties their bowels in a diaper? Our Creator did not design us for this function to be unpleasant.

Jenny and I are not into feces, or scat, as it is sometimes called. Jenny and I are fastidiousness in matters of personal hygiene.

I have a strong feeling that my use of enemas and colonic irrigation make my prostate and overall sexual function stronger. Jenny thinks enemas have enhanced our sex lives from the beginning, from childhood to marriage, and I agree. We both know that what we think is good for us may be just the opposite for anyone else. Neither of us recommends enemas or colonic irrigation for others. We feel that a person should first see a qualified and licensed health professional.

Since our marriage, years ago we continue to have health exams, including colon inspections. We believe in

the benefits of having skilled, caring personal physicians. They are intelligent, knowledgeable people. They may not all agree with our use of enemas, but they are extremely important in our health care.

Mom and Fran helped encourage us to have colon exams from the very beginning of our marriage, especially me, out of caution that my IBS may be masking another health problem.

Over the years I have had several more barium x-rays to make sure my colon was healthy. The last preparation I had for the barium enema x-ray was not the enema, but swallowing about a gallon of special fluid the night before. The fluid cleaned me out, but made me horrendously ill. I am going to arrange for enemas or colonic irrigation next time. We also have submitted to a sigmoidoscope exam about every three years. The only preparation for that exam is to take two small disposable enemas at home before the exam, one right after the other. This is an office procedure. We usually lie on the left side, or on a special table that flips the patient onto his or her head, with butt up in the air. The doctor inserts a long, flexible scope deep into our colon and takes a look through a lighted scope. The scope goes almost up to where the colon bends over the top of the

abdomen. We both have been told that most colon troubles occur in the length examined by the sigmoidoscope. All of these examinations have resulted in the doctor saying our colons look very good. We went for an examination just a month ago. We were both declared to be healthy.

I have had another type of colon exam, a colonoscope. This was done in the hospital with mild sedation. I tried drinking the great volume of solution the night before as with the barium exam, but I had the same sick reaction. From now on, regardless of the type of test, I will take old-fashioned enemas or colonic irrigation.

The colonoscope procedure was done on my left side in a small operating room-like place. Cables and video monitors were everywhere. A rather large hose was inserted into my colon. It was also a scope exam where the doctor can get a close look at the interior of the colon. This is not just some small flexible tube like the sigmoidscope. This is larger sized. The scope is taken all the way around the bend at the top into the ascending colon on the right side. It was not terribly painful because they kept shooting me with a sedative. This is a major intrusion into the colon.

Later in his office, the doctor told me my colon looked great and was nice and healthy. He said that I had Irritable

Bowel Syndrome, something I had known for years. However, this doctor was a well- known specialist, and after such a thorough exam, I had a solid confirmation that I had IBS, and that nothing else was wrong. I learned that IBS is diagnosed by eliminating other diseases. How something like IBS can be so painful and debilitating, while at the same time being relatively harmless, is a mystery to me. But that diagnosis is a good one to have, compared to the many morbid alternatives.

So with all of these tests and inspections of our colons, we are reasonably sure enemas or colonic irrigations have not been harmful to either of us. We tend to believe the enemas and colonic irrigations have brought us better health. For me, they are part of a regimen that allows me to live an almost normal life. With the steps that I take, I rarely have an acute spastic-colon attack. We also believe that enemas have helped us when we have been sick, and hastened our recuperation. We also believe they have prevented illness. We can not prove these statements scientifically, but we both feel that this inexpensive therapy will someday be proven very valuable when researched. Enemas have been used for thousands of years by many intelligent people with keen powers of observation. The

results of those observations made them believe good came from the practice. That certainly has been our experience as well.

About three years after our marriage, God blessed us with a child, David. Then, two years later, we had a little girl, Ruth, the apple of my eye. They were two of the cutest children on the planet. Fortunately, neither child inherited my IBS condition. They were unusually healthy. Jenny never allowed them to develop the atrocious eating habits of most children.

For the most part, enemas for them were replaced by what man had learned about diet since my birth. Although the enema and colonic irrigation played a limited role in both children's lives, they knew the business end of an enema bag at home, and a few times at their grandparents'. Ruth got food poisoning on a visit to their aunt Anna's, and she gave Ruth an enema with our permission, for which she was grateful.

Although David and Ruth received enemas when they stayed home from school sick, they were rarely sick. Like most very young children, they would be occasionally constipated, and Jenny would just bend them over her knee and give them a small bulb enema to easily and quickly

relieve the problem. Neither Jenny nor I can understand why many parents let their constipated children scream as they try to move their constipated bowels, potentially wreaking havoc upon the veins in their rectums. Equally foolish in our eyes was giving a child laxatives to irritate their whole gastrointestinal tract. Introducing children to enemas via the small bulb syringe was quick and simple, and not so scary. When they were older, about nine, Jenny gave them the larger bag enemas. By starting with the smaller bulb-enema syringe, and with Jenny's loving ways, there was nothing left for our children to fear. Our children were raised as we were regarding enemas, but with up-to-date dietary knowledge.

Jenny stayed at home until the kids were in school, then went back to teaching. This provided a perfect job for her and the family. Between the two of us, we were able to spend a great deal of time raising the children. When they were out after school, or home in the summer, Jenny was off work, too. Unlike many less fortunate parents, she knew what they were doing most of the time. She even knew their bowel habits, and could intervene when necessary. Many parents are so busy they do not know their children are on drugs, let alone their bowel habits.

As for Jenny and me, the enema provided a platform for "the talk." The only difference was we did not wait for one of them to have an orgasm or "wet dream." We advanced the idea by giving several small talks, starting when the children were much younger. This was better yet, and eliminated any potential emotional concerns by David or Ruth well in advance of things happening that they did not understand. I especially did not want David or Ruth to suffer any emotional distress due to masturbation, or even spontaneous ejaculation while receiving an enema. This also set the ground work to eliminate any embarrassment regarding sex later on. Although my emotional suffering due to ejaculation and my first self-administered enemas was short, the early talks with David and Ruth eliminated the possibilities of any such distress due to their not understanding their bodies. Emotional distress over anything is especially difficult at those early ages. I do not know when David or Jenny first masturbated, but when they did they understood it was a natural and normal event. The same was true of "wet dreams" and Ruth's first period.

We also explained to both children that they may be anally erotic, and the possible reasons why. We did not want them to be distressed if it turned out they were. A

significant portion of the world's population is anally erotic, and it is not cause for maladjustment.

At the same time we stressed that these matters were very personal and private. Jenny and I believe that enemas help awaken the anal nerves that we all have. We also explained that the children may, at some point, want to self-administer an enema, and that was okay as long as they were ready and did so properly. We wanted to make sure they understood that we were willing to help them to any extent needed. At the same time we wanted them to know that our giving them enemas was nothing to be embarrassed about, even though they may feel good.

Soon into puberty, and during the administration of an enema, Jenny briefly showed David where his prostate was, which allowed him to understand why an enema might feel good, and for him to better understand his sexual self.

In their teens, our children were given few enemas at home, but, rather, paid seasonal visits to our colon therapist. Like the ancient Egyptians, we believe the internal baths were the reason for their beautiful complexions.

Jenny and I both owe so much to our own families for setting us onto the road to good health. And I will never

forget my dear Doris and her love. All of the love we received enabled us to be even more open with our children, much to their benefit. David and Ruth grew up to be healthy, happy, loving, well-adjusted, and sweet people, just like my beloved partner for life-JENNY.

The End

Your Story

The author has found writing to be a healthy pursuit. It also makes him feel good to think that he may be helping another through what the author writes. Plus, it interesting and fun. You do not have to sell one book to win. Here is some space for some notes, an outline, or for a short story of your own. Give it a try. You may surprise yourself.

About the Author

The author has experienced a full range of blessings in life which include: a loving and full childhood with outstanding parents, college and legal educations, a successful business and professional life, a wonderful marriage with children, and last but certainly not least, good health.

He has also been through the *school of hard knocks,* where he learned the most, especially his appreciation of life itself.

He considers himself now blessed with the opportunity to write. He creates from the perspective that among the great gifts that our Creator most often gives man is health, which includes our sexuality. The author feels that the gift of health requires responsible care of and use of the body early on. The author views himself as looking at life through a set of clean eyes, which allows him to see our souls and bodies with a sense of wondrous beauty. He knows that this perspective is contrary to how some are socialized, but it feels right for him.

Printed in the United States
88590LV00001B/30/A